"*Systemic Diagnosis* is a must read for family therapy practitioners. In pointing out the flaws in other diagnostic models, Priest shows how theory-driven diagnosis sets the stage for effective systemic intervention. This book demonstrates each step of the systemic diagnosis model and equips readers to use it in their own practice. With great examples and guided practice, Priest makes difficult concepts easy to comprehend. The icing on the cake is that Priest writes like he's talking to a good friend, making it incredibly engaging. Five stars for this much needed book!"

Rebecca A. Cobb, PhD, LMFT, *Associate Clinical Professor and Clinical Coordinator, Couples and Family Therapy, Seattle University*

"*Systemic Diagnosis: An Application of Family Systems Theory* is a strongly recommended reading for all family therapists. Jacob Priest gives the reader a rich and thorough presentation of the possibilities and difficulties with the diagnosis systems at the same time as he suggests a systemic diagnosis system, rooted in family systems theory. The way systemic theory is transcended into the field of diagnosis is masterfully done. A presentation for the next generation of therapist."

Lennart Lorås, *Professor, Western Norway University of Applied Science and VID Spezialized University, Oslo-Norway*

Systemic Diagnosis

Systemic Diagnosis: An Application of Family Systems Theory helps marriage and family therapists incorporate theory-driven assessment and diagnosis into their practice, demonstrating how they can diagnose systems, not just individuals.

This introductory textbook argues that theory and diagnosis are key to providing excellent care in family therapy. Rooted in family systems theory, Jacob B. Priest offers readers a model to diagnose the history, structure, and boundaries of family systems. Chapters begin by looking at traditional and relational models of diagnosis before diving into systemic diagnosis. Readers are introduced to the EPIC assessment and guided on how to use it in their practice. Filled with case studies throughout, the book also includes digital content so students can practice a diagnosis process rooted in family systems theory.

Designed to be used on COAMFTE accredited programs, this book is essential for couple and family therapy students who are taking courses in assessment and mental health diagnosis and treatment.

Jacob B. Priest, PhD LMFT is an associate professor in the departments of Psychological and Quantitative Foundations, Internal Medicine – General Internal Medication, and Psychiatry, University of Iowa, USA.

Systemic Diagnosis
The Application of Family Systems Theory

Jacob B. Priest, PhD LMFT

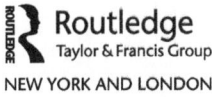

Routledge
Taylor & Francis Group

NEW YORK AND LONDON

Cover image: © Getty Image

First published 2024
by Routledge
605 Third Avenue, New York, NY 10158

and by Routledge
4 Park Square, Milton Park, Abingdon, Oxon, OX14 4RN

*Routledge is an imprint of the Taylor & Francis Group,
an informa business*

Library of Congress Cataloging-in-Publication Data
Names: Priest, Jacob Bird, author.
Title: Systemic diagnosis : the application of family systems
    theory / Jacob B. Priest, PhD LMFT.
Description: New York, NY : Routledge, 2024. | Includes
    bibliographical references and index.
Identifiers: LCCN 2023010794 (print) | LCCN 2023010795
    (ebook) | ISBN 9781032282480 (hardback) |
    ISBN 9781032282473 (paperback) | ISBN 9781003295907
    (ebook)
Subjects: LCSH: Systemic therapy (Family therapy)
Classification: LCC RC488.5 .P753 2024 (print) | LCC RC488.5
    (ebook) | DDC 616.89/156—dc23/eng/20230526
LC record available at https://lccn.loc.gov/2023010794
LC ebook record available at https://lccn.loc.gov/2023010795

ISBN: 978-1-032-28248-0 (hbk)
ISBN: 978-1-032-28247-3 (pbk)
ISBN: 978-1-003-29590-7 (ebk)

DOI: 10.4324/9781003295907

Typeset in Sabon
by Apex CoVantage, LLC

Access the Support Material: www.routledge.com/9781032282480

To Afton Elaine Bird and Birdie Afton Priest

Contents

Acknowledgements

Much of this book was written during the global COVID-19 pandemic, before and after the birth of my daughter, while moving to a new home, and while making the impossible decision to close the University of Iowa's couple and family therapy program. It wouldn't have happened without the patience and support of Heather Evans, my Editor at Routledge, my students, Kayla Reed-Fitzke, the University of Iowa libraries, and my wife, Chelsea.

Part I

Models of Diagnosis

I'll never forget one of my first experiences being a supervisor. I was running a supervision group with couple and family therapy PhD students at the University of Iowa. A student of mine was presenting about a family she was seeing. She provided the basic information about the family – the age of the parents and children, what brought them to therapy, and what their goals were. I followed up on the information she provided with what I thought was a logical question.

I asked, "How would you diagnose this family?"

Someone in the group replied, "As family therapists, we don't *believe* in diagnosis."

The response stunned me a bit, but as I looked around the room, the rest of the students were nodding. It seemed that they all agreed that providing a diagnosis to one or multiple members of the family wasn't systemic. As I dug deeper, many of them thought that diagnosing was something that they *had* to do, but it represented buying in to a model of care that was the antithesis of how family therapists are trained.

I stunned them a bit, when I replied, "I think diagnosis is essential to good family therapy."

I don't think disdain for diagnosis is limited to my students. Many couple and family therapists see diagnosis as problematic, and with good reason. Research has shown the most practiced model of diagnosis, the medical model, has lots of problems (National Academy of Sciences, Engineering, and Medicine, 2015). The issues with the medical model of diagnosis have led to conversations in many disciplines regarding the practice of diagnosis. Many in the mental health field are having ongoing debates about the problems with the current models of diagnosis, how to improve it, and what the future of diagnosis should look like (Hayes & Hofmann, 2020).

Yet, I don't see this debate happening within family therapy. It appears we have decided to opt out of the debate, leaving it to the psychologists and psychiatrists. It's almost as if we have implicitly decided that

DOI: 10.4324/9781003295907-1

whatever they decide on, we will begrudgingly accept, teach it to our students, apply it to our clients, and still talk about how diagnosis is not systemic.

But what if we could use family systems theory to create a model of diagnosis that was systemic? What if, instead of complaining about diagnosis, we used it to improve our practice? To improve our family therapy models? To improve our understanding of families?

I think systemic diagnosis can do all of this and more. But until family therapists begin to embrace diagnosis, understand how it's essential to good practice, and become experts in it, we are going to become like some of our clients – complaining but not yet willing to change. What's more, I think that unless and until we become experts in diagnosis, especially systemic diagnosis, we are going to be left out of the mainstream of psychotherapy practice – risking the future of our profession.

This book is about diagnosis – how it's typically done, and how it can be done better. This book is about how diagnosis as we currently understand it came to be and where it might go in the future. This book is about presenting a family systems theory model of diagnosis and demonstrating how it could be used in the therapy room.

This book is also an argument. It's an argument *against* the mainstream practice of diagnosis, and an argument *for* systemic diagnosis. It's an argument *against* family therapists who hold the idea that we "don't *believe* in diagnosis," and an argument *for* the idea that "diagnosis is essential to good family therapy."

Good arguments only happen when we are clear on what we are arguing about. So, let's start by clarifying certain ideas. As you'll notice, I've begun differentiating two models that inform diagnosis: the medical model and a systemic model. The distinction between these two models is important and the basis for the arguments I'm making throughout the book. But family therapists also need to be familiar with another idea: *relational* diagnosis. Some of you reading this may be familiar with this term – it's something the family therapists have been discussing for decades. I see diagnosis, relational diagnosis, and systemic diagnosis as having important differences. To make the case for why systemic diagnosis is important, we need to all be on the same page about the distinctions between these three models of diagnosis.

The goal of Part I of this book is to familiarize you with the traditional and relational models of diagnosis. Chapter 1 is about the most practiced model of diagnosis – diagnosis based on the medical model. I'll walk you through the medical model and how it has been applied to mental health disorders. I'll provide a case example of how clinicians would go about gathering the necessary information to make a diagnosis, and evaluate that diagnosis based on treatment response. After this, I'll walk through what I see and what research suggests are the drawbacks of traditional diagnosis. I'll talk briefly about some of the ideas that psychologists and psychiatrists are proposing to rectify the current issue with this model of diagnosis – especially when it comes to mental health disorders.

Chapter 2 is about relational diagnosis. The model of relational diagnosis has been around for some time – marriage and family therapists began advocating for it in the 1970s. In Chapter 2, I'll trace the history and development of relational diagnosis. I'll talk about the successes that the model has had addressing some of the limitations of traditional diagnosis and summarize some of the current research regarding the validity of the approach. A case example of how this model is applied is given, and I'll argue that while relational diagnosis is important, it's insufficient – at least when it comes to effective family therapy practice.

Chapter 1

The Medical Model of Diagnosis

For the last seven years, I've worked with psychiatrists who are in their third year of medical residency. During their third year, they come to the clinic, where I am the director, to learn how to do psychotherapy. While these residents tend to be novices when it comes to doing therapy, they excel in making diagnoses.

Unlike many family therapists, these third-year residents have spent years training to try to make accurate diagnoses. By the time they come to my clinic, they have studied diagnosis during medical school, and have had two years working in inpatient and outpatient psychiatry. Often, they are required to make an initial diagnosis and set a course of treatment within a 30-to-45-minute appointment. Their ability to diagnose mental health disorders exceeds that of many of my family therapy PhD students and many clinicians working in the field. When I ask these psychiatry residents about diagnosis and how they got proficient, they talk about the rigor of their training – training rooted in the medical model and the Diagnostic and Statistical Manual of Mental Disorders (DSM).

I've heard many family therapists use the phrase "medical model" to critique the process of diagnosis that psychiatrists and others use. But, when I ask them to define the medical model, they don't do it very well. So, that's where I want to start in this chapter – discussing the medical model. Without the understanding of the medical model, it's difficult to understand the diagnostic process, or the classification of diagnoses found in the DSM. If family therapists are going to critique the medical model used by psychiatrists and psychologists to create the diagnoses of the DSM, we need to be clear about what it is.

The Medical Model

What do we mean by the medical model? That depends on who you ask.

When most people talk about the medical model, they really are talking about the biomedical model. To me, the clearest definition of the biomedical model comes from one of its biggest critics, George Engel.

DOI: 10.4324/9781003295907-2

In 1977, Engel wrote an article titled, "The Need for a New Medical Model: A Challenge for Biomedicine." In it, Engel writes:

> The dominate model of disease today is biomedical, with molecular biology its basic scientific discipline. It assumes disease to be fully accounted for by deviations from the norm of measurable biological variables. . . . The biomedical model was devised by medical scientists for the study of disease. As such it was a scientific model; that is, it involved a shared set of assumptions and rules of conduct based on the scientific method and constituted a blueprint for research.

Engel's definition is often what family therapists and other mental healthcare providers think about when discussing the medical model. The medical model, as they understand it, assumes that all health problems are biological problems. If we can change the biological variables, then we can change the problem.

Engel saw many problems with the biomedical model. But his main issue with it resided in what is known as reductionism and mind-body dualism:

> The biomedical model not only requires that disease be dealt with as an entity independent of social behavior, it also demands that behavioral aberrations be explained on the basis of disordered (biochemical or neurophysiological) process. Thus the biomedical model embraces both reductionism, the philosophic view that complex phenomena are ultimately derived from a single primary principle, and mind-body dualism, the doctrine the separates the mental from the somatic.

In Engel's view, the biomedical model focused too narrowly. He wasn't arguing that we abandon the exploration of the biological causes of disease, but that social behavior is important as is recognizing connections between the mind and body.

Engel rooted his critique and his proposal of a better model, the biopsychosocial model, in systems theory. Drawing on the work of Ludwig Von Bertalanffy, Engel argued the doctors needed to ground their work in systems theory. He argued that systems theory:

> by treating sets of related events collectively as systems manifesting functions and properties on the specific level of the whole, has made possible recognition of isomorphies across different levels of organization, as molecules, cells, organs, the organism, the person,

the family, the society, or the biosphere. From such isomorphies can be developed fundamental laws and principles that operate commonly at all levels of organization, as compared to those which are unique for each. Since systems theory holds that all levels of organization are linked to each other in a hierarchical relationship so that change in one affects change in the others, its adoption as a scientific approach should do much to mitigate the holist-reductionist dichotomy.

In other words, if we can view diseases, whether mental or physical, as part of interconnecting systems we can better understand them. What's more, he is arguing that by using systems theory we might be able to look at similarities across systems and find ways to describe the "why, what for, as well as how?" (p. 134) of the disease process.

Many have pushed back on Engel's critique. Premal Shah and Deborah Mountain (2007) argued that Engel and others had mispresented what is meant by the medical model and suggested that with the correct definition, the medical model would be readily adopted. In their article title, "The Medical Model Is Dead – Long Live the Medical Model," they wrote:

> We believe that we need a simple definition of the medical model, which incorporates medicine's fundamental ideals, to facilitate clarity and precision, without denying its shortcomings. We propose that the 'medical model' is the process whereby, informed by the best available evidence, doctors advise on, coordinate or deliver interventions for health improvement. It can be summarily stated as 'does it work?'

Put simply the medical model is a process that a doctor uses to identify clinical problems. If they identify the problem accurately, they should be able to intervene effectively. If the intervention is effective, it should "work" – alleviate the presenting problem of the patient. If it doesn't work, the process starts over again.

A similar definition of the medical model was given by Ahmed Samei Huda in his book, *The Medical Model in Mental Health: An Explanation and Evaluation* (2019). He writes that the medical model:

> involves assessing a patient, then making decisions and interventions based on this assessment, followed by monitoring the response to these interventions by further assessments which may lead to changes in decision and interventions, and so on in a cycle of assessment/ interventions/assessment of the effect of interventions and changes

in severity. These assessments are undertaken principally by talking to the patients in order to acquire a medical history but also by performing a clinical examination, ordering any relevant tests, and seeking additional details such as information from relatives and/or carers.

The doctor then uses this information to make diagnosis (or more than one diagnosis). They also incorporate other important information into a 'diagnostic formulation,' and decide on a management plan that incorporates discussing with the patient the likely range of outcomes and the choice of recommended further treatments and further investigations.

Like Shah and Mountain, Huda argues that the medical model is the process that results in diagnosis, intervention, and continued assessment.

Huda also talks about the biomedical model pointing out how critiques, like the one discussed by Engel earlier, are incorrect. He writes:

> People often refer to the 'biomedical model' and sometimes understand this incorrectly to mean a model that focuses exclusively on a person's biology and biological interventions. The biomedical model also integrates the effects of culture, social factors, personal circumstances and beliefs, diet, upbringing, and so forth on health and illness. It can even accommodate the notion that psychological or social factors may be more important in the causation of certain conditions than biological factors and that the best intervention is not necessarily biological (e.g. medication) and often involves interventions based on psychological or social factors. However, the biomedical model tends to view non-biological factors' effect on health as due to their effect on an intermediate biological factor.

Here, Huda makes the case that the medical model also isn't a "disease based model." He suggests that this misunderstanding stems from the idea that a medical diagnosis refers to distinct disease and is not related to other diagnoses, biological processes, or psychosocial factors.

Many would read what Huda is suggesting and argue that it is exactly what Engel proposed as a biopsychosocial model. However, as Sarah Woods (2019) points out, there is an important distinction between what Huda describes and Engel's view of a biopsychosocial model. She writes:

> Engel cited general systems theory as a conceptual road map for the field of medicine to use to consider both the study of disease and the medical care required to treat it. . . . Engel stressed that an illness, an

individual, a family, and their social context are all parts of a larger whole, critical to understanding health and health care. . . . Engel specified the hierarchical levels in which each individual is embedded. The hierarchy begins at the level of subatomic particles and extends to the biosphere, with the individual embedded as the highest level of the organismic hierarchy, and as the lowest levels of the social hierarchy. Each level of the hierarchy is distinct, 'an organized dynamic whole,' and at the same time, embedded within and influenced by higher levels.

The distinction between what Huda is saying and what Engel and Woods are saying seems small, but I'd argue that it's large. Huda talks about "factors" while Woods and Engel talk about "systems." A system has interactions and purpose. A factor is a circumstance that might influence something. A system is dynamic, reciprocal, and adaptive. A factor is linear and static. Systems can tell us why and how, and systems-based explanations can account for multiple causes. Factors only provide us with correlations and associations, and often do a poor job telling us why or how.

This distinction is important, and as you'll see, key to the central argument of this book. We'll be returning to this distinction many times throughout this book. But for now, I want to be clear about how I am distinguishing these terms. When I talk about the medical model, I'm referring to the process of intervention. When I talk about biomedical or biopsychosocial models, I'm talking about models that have ideological differences in what contributes to disease and to health.

Diagnosis and the Diagnostic Process

Now that I've spelled out what I see as the distinction between the medical, biomedical, and biopsychosocial model, I want to shift to a related idea: diagnosis. Diagnosis and the diagnosis process are embedded in the models I've discussed earlier. To intervene effectively, or to "do what works," you need to diagnose well. To diagnose well you need to know what causes disease and what contributes to health. The way you diagnose depends on what you see contributes to disease and health. And to determine if something works, you must determine what needs to change. None of that is possible without diagnosis.

Most of this book is going to focus on diagnosis of mental health disorders – that's the realm in which family therapists work and get paid. But to start, I want to talk about diagnosis more broadly. Diagnosis and diagnoses as discussed in the DSM have roots in the broader process of medical diagnosis.

In 2015, the National Academies of Sciences, Engineering, and Medicine published the results of a study of diagnosis. In framing this study, the researchers defined diagnosis as follows:

> Diagnosis has been described as both a process and a classification scheme, or a 'pre-existing set of categories agreed upon by the medical profession to designate a specific condition' (Jutel, 2009). When a diagnosis is accurate and made in a timely manner, clinical decision making will be tailored to a correct understanding of the patient's health problem.

As they describe, diagnosis is about classification and categorization. Scientists and practitioners come together and, based on research and clinical experience, designate clusters of symptoms to reflect a specific condition. If a patient goes to the hospital and they report feeling sad, report changes in their sleeping patterns, have thoughts of suicide, and have lost interest in things that used to bring them joy, this cluster of symptoms will most likely be labeled "depression."

Along with providing a definition of *diagnosis*, the researchers from the National Academies of Science, Engineering, and Medicine also define the term "diagnostic process." They define diagnostic process as:

> a complex, patient-centered, collaborative activity that involves information gathering and clinical reasoning with the goal of determining a patient's health problem. This process occurs over time, within the context of a larger health care work system that influences the diagnostic process.

Expanding on this definition, they provided what they see as steps of the diagnosis process as follows:

> First, a patient experiences a health problem. The patient is likely the first person to consider his or her symptoms and may choose at this point to engage with the health care system. Once a patient seeks health care, there is an iterative process of information gathering, information integration and interpretation, and determining a working diagnosis. Performing a clinical history and interview, conducting a physical exam, performing diagnostic testing, and referring or consulting with other clinicians are all ways of accumulating information that may be relevant to understanding a patient's health problem. The information gathering approaches can be employed at different times, and diagnostic information can be obtained in different orders. The continuous process of information gathering, integration, and interpretation involves hypothesis generation and

updating prior probabilities as more information is learned. Communication among health professionals, the patient, and the patient's family is critical in this cycle of information gathering.

The end goal of the diagnostic process is to create a working diagnosis. A working diagnosis is a list of one or more potential diagnoses that are communicated to the patient and are used to plan a course of treatment. It's called a working diagnosis because as more information is gathered through assessment and treatment, the diagnosis may change. The accuracy of a working diagnosis is evaluated through patient outcomes. If the patient responds to treatment well, it's likely one or more of your working diagnoses were the correct diagnoses. If the patient doesn't respond, this means more information is needed to improve the diagnosis or to improve treatment.

Diagnosis and the diagnostic process described here are typically rooted in the biomedical model. When doctors think about disease, they are typically focusing on biological variables. This is evidenced in the treatment prescribed. If someone goes to the doctor and they get diagnosed with diabetes, they will often be prescribed medication, a change in diet, and exercise. This intervention assumes that the issue resides within the biological systems of the individual. And we would determine that the diagnosis is correct if we see changes in these biological systems after a certain amount of time using medication, changing the diet, and doing continuous exercise. In other words, if the symptoms can be identified and treated, then the diagnostic process was successful, the diagnosis was accurate, and the problem is alleviated.

But does this work? Remember the medical model means "doing what works." If we are diagnosing well, administering the correct treatments, then people should get better. If this process of diagnosis centered in the biomedical model works, then we should have evidence that people are getting better. And for our purposes here, if the diagnosis process works in mental health, we should have strong evidence for reliability in creating diagnoses and good treatment outcomes. But before we examine the evidence, I want to provide an example of how the diagnosis of mental health disorders typically takes place. No two providers diagnose in the same way. But when it comes to mental health disorders, we are often all beholden to the same book – The Diagnostic and Statistical Manual of Mental Disorders (DSM) – at least in the United States.

Diagnosis and the DSM

If you're reading this book, I'm guessing that you're at least somewhat familiar with the DSM. If you're a practicing therapist, it's likely you have a copy of at least one version of the DSM somewhere in your office. If you're a family therapy student, you'll eventually own a copy. The DSM is currently in its fifth, and many have suggested, last edition. It's a book that stokes lots of controversy and is at the center of the debate around diagnosis. To understand the DSM in its current form, how it is used to create diagnoses, and the debate about it, you need to understand its origins. So, let's start there.

The first know classification of mental health disorders in the United States was created by the National Committee for Mental Health Hygiene in 1918. This manual, called the Statistical Manual for the Use of Institutions for the Insane, contained 22 major diagnostic categories. These categories were mostly focused on things that were understood to have a biological origin – alcohol use, brain trauma, etc. Only one of the categories, "psychoneuroses and neuroses," was believed to be "psychogenic in nature." This manual underwent ten revisions between 1918 and 1940. But just about the time of World War II, the process of psychiatry in the United States changed radically (Clegg, 2012).

The large number of soldiers who experienced war related trauma during World War II led to a rethinking of the classification of mental disorders. As Joshua Clegg described it:

> a large number of psychiatrists involved in treating war related psychological trauma found success in applying psychodynamic therapy to psychogenetic disorders and, as a result, these clinicians became dissatisfied with the existing biological oriented, symptom-based classification system. One expression of this disaffection was the formation of a committee from the Office of the Surgeon General, chaired by Brigadier General William C. Menninger, the goal of which was to produce an alternative classification scheme. The document produced by this committee, called *Medical 203* adopted a new way of classifying psychopathology.

This new classification scheme conceptualized psychopathology as a response to multiple distressing circumstances instead of biological problems with biological origins. Medical 203 had ten basic diagnostic categories. These included grouping such as "Simple Personality Reactions," "Character and Behavior Disorders," "Immaturity Reactions," and "Affective Disorders."

Though Medical 203 was probably the most well-known diagnostic manual in circulation in the early 1900s, there were also many others. Part of the reason DSM-I was developed was to try and consolidate the many classification schemes. In the 1952 foreword of DSM-I, George Raines noted:

> The development of a uniform nomenclature of disease in the United States is comparatively recent. In the late [1920s], each large teaching

center employed its own origination, no one of which met more than the immediate needs of local institutions. Despite their local origins, for the lack of suitable alternatives, these systems were spread in use throughout the nation, ordinarily by individuals who had been trained in a particular center, hence had become accustomed to that special system of nomenclature. Modifications in the transplanted nomenclatures immediately became necessary, and were made as expediency dictated. There resulted a polyglot of diagnostic labels and systems, effectively blocking communication and the collection of medical statistics.

Raines argued that if mental health work was going to advance, it needed to be standardized. That way, regardless of training location, everyone would use the same system, resulting in a better idea of patterns of mental health across the country.

DSM-I maintained the psychodynamic language that was found in Medical 203 and had many similar categorizations. These groupings included "Disorders Caused by or Associated with Impairment of Brain Tissue Function," "Mental Deficiency," and "Disorders of Psychogenic Origin or Without Clearly Defined Physical Cause or Structural Change in the Brain." The authors of DSM-I argued that all mental disorders could be divided into two major groups:

1) those in which there is disturbance of mental function resulting from, or precipitated by, a primary impairment of the function of the brain, generally due to diffuse impairment of brain tissue; and 2) those which are the result of more general difficulty in adaption of the individual, and in which any associated brain function disturbance is secondary to the psychiatric disorder.

DSM-II was published in 1968. This iteration of the DSM was in part developed in response to the publication of the World Health Organization's eighth addition of the international classification of diseases (ICD-8) that was published in 1966. The foreword of the DSM-II, written by Ernest Gruenberg, outlines the distinction between it and the ICD-8 and DSM-I. He wrote:

The second edition of the Diagnostic and Statistical Manual of Mental Disorders reflects the growth of the concept that people of all nations live in one world. . . . In preparing this Manual the Committee had to make adjustments within a few of the ICD categories to make them better conform to U.S. usage. . . . In publishing the Manual the Association provides a service to the psychiatrists of the United States and presents a nomenclature that is usable in mental hospitals, psychiatric units, and in office practice. . . . The first edition of this Manual (1952) made an important contribution to the U.S. and, indeed, world psychiatry. It was reprinted twenty times through 1967 and distributed widely in the U.S. and other countries. . . . In preparing this new edition, the Committee has been particularly conscious of its usefulness in helping stabilize nomenclature in textbook and professional literature.

Though there were some changes from DSM-I to DSM-II, DSM-II was still rooted in psychodynamic thought. DSM-II notably added sections on childhood disorders and dropped the term "reaction" from its description. But many of the changes were minor compared to the shift that occurred between DSM-II and DSM-III (Clegg, 2012).

DSM-III represented a profound shift in the classification of mental disorders. While DSM-I and II drifted away from the biomedical model, DSM-III was rooted firmly in it. As Joshua Clegg noted:

> The remedicalization of the DSM through the emphasis on diagnosis formed a core guiding principle of DSM-III. . . . DSM-III also attempted to remove all evidence of early psychodynamic explanations for mental disorders and, instead, reframed diagnostic categories according to symptom clusters or patterns. . . . The removal of explicitly theoretical descriptions left DSM-III without any clear basis for the diagnostic categories provided, other than the consensus of clinical judgment, the framers of the manual considered empirical evidence to be the appropriate check on the idiosyncrasies of personal judgment: 'In attempting to resolve various diagnostic issues, the Task Force relied, as much as possible, on research evidence relevant to various kinds of diagnostic validity (p. 3).' This assertion reflected the growing belief that the diagnosis and treatment of mental disorders would have to be based on data.

The decision to move from a classification scheme based on theory to a "theory-neutral" classification scheme resulted mainly from what was seen as an attack on psychiatry. Joshua Clegg further noted:

> The antipsychiatry movement, including challenges from both professionals and patient advocacy groups, had gathered momentum, the psychodynamic approach at the root of the early DSMs was in decline, and the manual itself was under attack, both in terms of its lack of empirical validation and because of the certain controversial diagnostic categories (e.g., homosexuality).

DSM-III was rooted in the biomedical model of psychological disorders based on research. The committee that created DSM-III wanted their classification to be based on data relevant to diagnostic validity. Doing this, they argued, would allow for "empirical evidence to be the appropriate check on the idiosyncrasies of personal judgement (Clegg, 2012, p. 366)."

The next few iterations of the DSM (DSM-III-TR, DSM-IV, and DSM-IV-TR) were smaller. DSM-III-TR included some recategorization based on new evidence, including the additional "developmental disorders." The most significant addition in DSM-IV was the larger emphasis on cultural aspects of diagnosis. These included things such as cultural variations of diagnoses and ways to report the "cultural context" of a individual being diagnosis (Clegg, 2012). The aim of this edition was to make the DSM applicable across cultures. DSM-IV-TR was also published but with only minor changes.

At the time of this writing, the DSM is in its fifth iteration. What is in the DSM-5? It's a large book – it has 947 pages. The DSM-5 and its revision, the DSM-5-TR, has 20 diagnostic chapters. Within these 20 chapters there are 541 diagnostic categories, but only 151 categories are defined using diagnostic criteria (Blashfield et al., 2014). The introduction to DSM-5-TR suggests:

> The chapters in DSM-5 and DSM-5-TR are sequenced in recognition of the advances in our understanding of the underlying vulnerabilities and symptom characteristics of disorders. This sequence reflects what has been learned during the past decades about how the brain functions and how genes and environment influence a person's health and behavior.
>
> The chapters are also grouped by broad categories that – in some cases – indicate the common features within larger disorder groups. . . . DSM-5 and DSM-5-TR are organized in sequence with the developmental lifespan. This organization is evident in every chapter and within individual diagnostic categories, with disorders typically diagnosed in childhood detailed first, followed by those in adolescence, adulthood, and later life.

I'm not going to spend time talking about each chapter or each diagnosis – that's what the DSM is for. Instead, I'm going to assume that you are at least somewhat familiar with the contents of the DSM to demonstrate how you might make a diagnosis. If you're not, I'd suggest you spend some time getting familiar with it before going forward.

Making a DSM-5 Diagnosis

What's the process of making a diagnosis based on DSM-5? I want to provide an example. If you're familiar with this process, you can probably skip this next section, but if you aren't or if you want a review, I'm going to walk you through how a diagnosis might be made.

To demonstrate the process of diagnosis based on what's in the DSM-5, let me introduce you to Dave. Dave is a 23-year-old cis-gender white male. Let's pretend that Dave comes into my therapy office because he's been feeling "really stressed out." Dave lives in Iowa. He graduated from trade school about a year ago and has been working as an electrician. He's close to his family, especially his mom. He's single, but he has been using dating apps to try and meet people. What follows is a hypothetical conversation between Dave and me. The purpose of this conversation is to diagnose Dave using the criteria found in DSM-5.

As you'll see, Dave is going to end up with a diagnosis of generalized anxiety disorder (GAD). The DSM-5 diagnostic criteria for GAD are as follows:

1. Excessive anxiety and worry (apprehension expectation), occurring more days than not for at least six months, about a number of events or activities (such as school or work performance).
2. The person finds it difficult to control the worry.
3. The anxiety and worry are associated with three or more of the following six symptoms (with at least some symptoms present for more days than not for the past six months) – restlessness or feeling keyed up or on edge; being easily fatigued; difficulty concentrating or mind going blank; irritability; muscle tension; and/or sleep disturbance (difficulty falling or staying asleep, or restless unsatisfying sleep).
4. The disturbance is not better explained by another mental disorder (e.g., anxiety or worry about having panic attacks in panic disorder, negative evaluation in social anxiety disorder [social phobia], contamination or other obsessions in obsessive-compulsive disorder, separation from attachment figures in separation anxiety disorder, reminders of traumatic events in posttraumatic stress disorder, gaining weight in anorexia nervosa, physical complaints in somatic symptom disorder, perceived appearance flaws in body dysmorphic disorder, having a serious illness in illness anxiety disorder, or the content of delusional beliefs in schizophrenia or delusional disorder).
5. The anxiety, worry, or physical symptoms cause clinically significant distress or impairment in social, occupational, or other important areas of functioning.
6. The disturbance is not due to the direct physiological effects of a substance (e.g., a drug of abuse, a medication) or a general medical condition (e.g., hyperthyroidism) and does not occur exclusively during a mood disorder, a psychotic disorder, or a pervasive developmental disorder.

In this conversation with Dave, I'm going to start with the symptoms he's presenting with, I'm going to assess for other symptoms that could rule out other diagnoses, and then I'm going to drill down specifically on the criteria related to GAD. This conversation is going to be straightforward. Often the process of making a diagnosis isn't as clean. But I'm hoping in reading this, you can get a sense for the major aims of our conversation.

Therapist: Hi, Dave. Thanks for making it today. My name is Jacob, and today I'm going to ask you some questions to help us get a better understanding of what's been going on. Okay? This is what we tend to call an initial assessment. My questions are going to be really general to start out but will get more specific eventually. Does that sound alright?

Dave: Yeah. Sounds good.

Therapist: Great. Also, if any of the questions I ask make you feel uncomfortable or bring up something you'd rather not talk about, that's okay. You don't have to answer any question that you don't want to.

Dave: Ok.

Therapist: So in the paperwork you completed, you said that you were feeling stressed out? Is that right?

Dave: Yeah.

Therapist: Can you tell me a bit more about that? What's been stressing you out?

Dave: Well, work has been super busy lately. My boss has been on my ass to get jobs done quickly, but I've only been doing this a year, so sometimes I run into things that I haven't dealt with before.

Therapist: That does sound stressful. Is your work your main source of stress or are there other things going on as well?

Dave: Work is what's making the most stress, yeah, but you know the other things have been stressing me out too. Typical stuff – bills, family shit, that kind of stuff. But it's just been more than usual.

Therapist: Okay. So is this level of stress different than your normal stress?

Dave: Yeah.

Therapist: How so?

Dave: Like, normally when I'm stressed I can deal. Go to the bar with friends, watch the game. Maybe hit the gym. But lately, I can't seem to let go of it.

Therapist: The stress?

Dave: Yeah. It's like my brain won't turn off.

Therapist: And this is unusual, yeah? Have you ever felt like this before?

Dave: No, not really. I mean, like I said, typically I can deal with stress, but this is different.

Therapist: And how long has this kind of stress being going on? A week? A few months? Longer?

Dave: I mean, I think a few months. My mom says I've been different since like Christmas.

Therapist: So, six months? How does your mom say you've been different?

Dave: Like on edge. She says I get mad more often and like I can't sit still for very long. She always tells me to calm down and that just pisses me off even more.

Therapist: And do you feel on edge like every day? Or a few times a week? Let's say during the past two weeks, how many days have you felt this kind of stress?

Dave: Hmm . . . probably like . . . well basically everyday. I mean, maybe there's days when like it's not as bad but most of the time, especially in the last week or two it's been bad.

Therapist: I'm sorry; that sounds difficult?

Dave: Yeah, it sucks.

Therapist: And does this stress come with feeling down or depressed?

Dave: Not really. It's mostly just being stressed out?

Therapist: So not really feelings down or hopeless?

Dave: No.

Therapist: Okay. And has this stress effected your sleep? Do you sleep less than usual or a lot more?

Dave: When I'm really stressed, it takes a while for my brain to shut off, so it's harder to fall asleep. But when I sleep, I sleep pretty good.

Therapist: Have you noticed having lots of additional energy? Or that you're starting lots of projects?

Dave: No, not really.

Therapist: Have you found yourself taking more risks than usual?

Dave: What do you mean?

Therapist: Like have you noticed like spending money on stuff that you typically wouldn't or doing things that are unnecessarily risky or over the top?

Dave: No. I mean sometimes I do stupid shit, but nothing too risky. I'm not like flying to Vegas to blow 5 grand on slots or anything.

Therapist: Do you find yourself avoiding places you'd typically go because of your stress? Or feeling panicked by going somewhere?

Dave: Well, I still go to work, hang with friends and whatnot. Sometimes I feel anxious going but I still go. I may have a hard time focusing when I'm there, but I'll still go.

Therapist: Okay. And when you go out with friends, what do you do?

Dave: I mean I will got to a bar to watch the game. Or maybe hang out at a friend's house.

Therapist: And how much might you drink when you go out?

Dave: I mean sometimes I drink too much. But I don't think it's an issue. You know, if we are watching a game, I'll probably knock back a few more than I should.

Therapist: How often would you say that you drink more than four drinks in day?

Dave: I mean maybe I'd do that on the weekend, but like I might have one beer a night during the week. I have to get up too early for work, so I can't go hard during the week.

Therapist: And when you drink do you smoke or take anything else?

Dave: I don't smoke – you mean cigarettes, right? No. Occasionally I'll smoke weed, but that's pretty rare. And other stuff like drugs?

Therapist: Yes. Drugs or pills?

Dave: No. I've seen that shit fuck too many people up.

Therapist: Alright. And when you feel stressed or anxious, do feel like people can hear your thoughts? Or that you could hear other people's thoughts?

Dave: No, not really. I mean, when I'm stressed I have like thoughts that replay over and over but like I don't think people can hear them or whatever.

Therapist: And do you ever hear things that other people don't hear, or see things they don't see?

Dave: You mean like in that movie? Ahh man, what's it called? With the guy from Gladiator? My mom really liked it growing up.

Therapist: A Beautiful Mind? Russell Crowe?

Dave: Yeah. I never liked it, but . . . no, nothing like that.

Therapist: Okay. And is there anything else that you feel or experience when your stressed?

Dave: Not really.

Therapist: Have you ever had thoughts of suicide? Or that you'd be better off dead?

Dave: No, for me it's not like that.

Therapist: Okay. Any problems with your memory? Or do you ever feel distant or detached from your body?

Dave: No, nothing like that.

Therapist: Mostly it's feeling anxious, on edge or irritated?

Dave: Yeah.

Therapist: And it's been going on pretty consistently for six months?

Dave: Yeah.

Therapist: And with this stress and anxiety have you ever felt panicked?

Dave: Like a panic attack?

Therapist: Yes.

Dave: No. My mom had those when I was growing up, but like I've never really had one. I mean sometimes I'll feel pretty overwhelmed but not like needing to go to the hospital like my mom did.

Therapist: And did this happen a lot with your mom?

Dave: Yeah, I mean not a ton, but I can remember times when she would be like super scared and couldn't breathe and stuff. My dad would take her to the ER, and she'd be fine. It probably happened a few times when I was younger.

Therapist: But you've never experienced that?

Dave: Nope.

Therapist: So when you feel stressed or anxious, is it about something in particular? Is there something you tend to worry about or feel like you don't have control over?

Dave: Like what?

Therapist: Like being embarrassed in public or being reminded of something that happened in the past, or maybe that you might be sick or have something wrong with your body?

Dave: No. My stress doesn't tend to be about one thing. You know, I might be stressed about work and not doing a good job one day. And the next day I'm feeling stressed because I feel like I can't focus on shit. Other days I'm just like tired from all the stress.

Therapist: Yeah, okay. And do you try to control the stress or the worry?

Dave: Yeah, but it doesn't work. I mean, I may be distracted from it by something but it comes back. And sometimes I feel like I can't control it at all and that it's always gonna be there.

Therapist: Have you talked to anyone about this before? Like a doctor?

Dave: Yeah, I went to a doctor first and they are the ones that sent me to you.

Therapist: So, what did that doctor say about your health?

Dave: I mean physically, she said I was doing good. I work out and stuff, so she wasn't concerned about like anything about that. She just wanted me to get some help for my stress.

Therapist: Got it. Was there anything else the doctor said or was concerned about?

Dave: She asked my about my drinking and stuff too, but she wasn't too worried.

Therapist: Okay, if I'm getting this right, it seems to me that for the last six months or so, you've been pretty stressed and worried. It's not really about one thing in particular, but it's worry that you have a hard time controlling?

Dave: Yeah.

Therapist: And this stress and worry make you feel tired? And on edge?

Dave: Yeah, I get pretty chippy too sometimes.

Therapist: Like irritable or like angry?

Dave: More like frustrated or irritable, I guess. I don't want to like fight with people, but I'm just not as go with the flow as I used to be.

Therapist: Okay. And you have trouble falling asleep because of the worry and stress?
Dave: Yeah.

As you can see from this conversation, Dave meets the criteria for GAD based on the criteria of the DSM-5. He has excessive worry and anxiety that has been occurring more days than not for at least six months. It's hard for him to control this worry and he describes feeling keyed up, and difficulty concentrating and sleeping. It appears Dave's anxiety isn't being caused by another medical issue or from the effect of substances such as alcohol or drugs.

Though this diagnosis describes and classifies what Dave is experiencing, it doesn't tell us why it's happening, how it developed, or why it keeps happening. Nor is that necessarily the purpose of the diagnoses of the DSM-5. The goal of the diagnoses in the DSM-5 is to provide doctors, therapists, and patients with common language to communicate about a group of symptoms. It tries to afford consistent and reliable diagnostic categories that researchers can study. Although the goal of the DSM-5 diagnoses isn't to recommend or provide treatment guidelines, they were created to provide an accurate diagnosis so that treatment can be effective.

Criticism of the DSM-5 and the Medical Model of Diagnosis

But how effective is the DSM-5 at providing consistent and reliable diagnoses? And does this type of diagnosis result in effective treatment? As I noted earlier, many people have criticized the DSM-5, and many of these criticisms have been validated by research. But, as you'll see, the issues of the DSM-5 may have been around for quite some time.

The DSM-5 and its revision, the DSM-5-TR, have been widely criticized for the lack of transparency in their development, for the weak methodology employed to make diagnostic changes, a failure to address the role of biology in mental illness, and the tie that many members of the committee had to the pharmaceutical industry (Bender et al., 2018; Cosgrove et al., 2006; Cuthbert & Insel, 2013). Edward Shorter (2015) summed up his criticisms of the DSM-5 as follows:

> It would be easy to think the DSM-5 evolved as a logical and scientific progression from DSM-IV. In fact, it evolved in a haphazard and politically driven manner from a century and a half of effort to get the classification of psychiatric illness right. In addition, the disappointing outcome of this entire endeavor is that, today the field's

> nosology seems even farther from . . . discerning the true illness of entities locked in the brain than . . . around 1900.

Shorter, like many others, is pretty disappointed with the current state of the DSM. And the evidence seems to support this.

In 2013, the results of a field trial evaluating the reliability of DSM-5 diagnoses were reported. These results came from 11 academic centers in the United States and Canada, and included 249 clinicians, and 2,246 patients, including both children and adults. To evaluate the reliability of the DSM-5 diagnoses, the researchers wanted to determine whether two clinicians would agree on the same diagnosis of a patient (Clarke et al., 2013). For most of the diagnoses tested, the researchers found what they described as good to very good reliability – meaning that when two clinicians evaluated the same patient, the probability that they would arrive at the same diagnoses was not due to chance. This value is known as kappa.

But others didn't agree with the interpretation of the kappa values that the researchers described. Allen Frances (2012), the chair of the DSM-IV taskforce, wildly criticized the methods, results, and conclusions of the field trial. Writing in the *Huffington Post*, Frances argued:

> "The whole purpose of having a manual of psychiatric diagnosis is to promote diagnostic agreement. . . . The results of the DSM-5 trials are a disgrace to the field. For context, in previous DSMs a diagnosis had to have a kappa reliability of about 0.6 or above to be considered acceptable. A reliability of 0.2 to 0.4 has always been considered completely unacceptable, not much above chance.

Frances notes that the researchers of the field trials found what he considered unacceptable kappa values for many of the major diagnoses (e.g., schizophrenia had a kappa of 0.46), and that these values were much lower than previous iterations of the DSM. For example, In the DSM-5 field trial, schizophrenia had a kappa of 0.46, while in the DSM-IV trial the kappa was 0.76. He argued:

> Reliability this low for so many diagnoses gravely undermines the credibility of the DSM-5 as a basis for administrative coding, treatment selection, and clinical research. . . . This assault on reliability was predicted, but its scope exceeds even my jaundiced fears and creates a DSM-5 emergency.

Others have suggested that this isn't just a problem of the DSM-5 and the reliability problem has existed in previous iterations of the DSM, specifically the DSM-IV that Allen Frances headed up. As Michael

Chmielewski and his colleagues (2015) noted, the DSM-5 field trial relied exclusively on the test-retest method (where two clinicians interviewed the same patient about a week apart). But in the trials for the DSM-IV, when reliability was assessed, it was done exclusively using audio recordings – one clinician would interview a client and another clinician would make a diagnosis based on that audio. They argued that the audio recording method may have inflated the reliability of the DSM-IV – meaning that the diagnostic categories have been problematic even before the DSM-5. They write:

> Although psychiatric diagnoses have become more reliable and valid since the publication of the DSM-III, the current results – together with those from the DSM-5 field trials – suggest that the reliability of psychological diagnosis may be lower than commonly believed. From this perspective, the DSM-5 field trials appear to have brought to light important issues regarding diagnostic reliability that have existed for some time but were obfuscated by common methods of assessing reliability. . . . Our results add to the large body of literature documenting the limitations of categorical diagnoses and indicate there is significant room for improvement.

In other words, the reliability of the DSM-5 categories isn't a new problem; it was one that was a part of DSM-IV, but it was hidden because of the methods.

The evidence seems to suggest that as currently constituted, the diagnostic categories aren't as reliable as the creator had hoped. But the goal of providing reliable diagnostic categories is to develop effective treatment. It may be that these categories are reliable enough to provide effective treatments. But is that the case? Let's look at the treatment outcomes of one of the common diagnoses of the DSM – major depressive disorder.

In 2020 Pim Cuijpers, Argyris Stringaris, and Miranda Wolpert summarized the current outcomes of depression treatment. Their survey of the research suggests that 54% of adults who take antidepressant medication experience a 50% reduction in symptoms; 35–40% of adults who take a placebo pill have a 50% reduction; and 53% of adults who didn't get treatment for depression also experienced symptom reduction after 12 months. What's more, 25–40% of adults who recover from depression will have another episode within two years, 60% will have another within five years, and 85% will have another within 15 years. In writing about the results, the authors allude to the reliability of the depression diagnosis. They write:

> Although many new refinements to treatments have been developed in the past decade, their efficacy has not improved over time.

Moreover, predicting who is most likely to benefit from which interventions or approaches is not currently possible. . . . Some of this is due to lack of clarity about what depression is, it's boundaries and possible heterogeneity.

When it comes to treatment for depression there is lots of room for improvement. Part of that improvement may come from how depression is categorized, or the boundaries around what is considered depression and what isn't.

To be fair, other DSM diagnoses have better outcomes. Treatment outcomes for anxiety disorders (e.g., social anxiety disorder [Cuijpers & van Straten, 2014], posttraumatic stress disorder [Kline et al., 2021], and generalized anxiety disorder [Baldwin et al., 2011]) are often better than that of depressive disorders. However, a problem with talking about the better outcomes for those with anxiety disorder is that many people who have anxiety disorders also have depression. As Ned Kangan summarized in 2020:

With respect to major depression, a worldwide survey reported that 45.7% of individuals with lifetime major depressive disorder had a lifetime history of one or more anxiety disorders. . . . From the perspective of anxiety disorders, the lifetime comorbidity of depression is estimated to range from 20% to 70% for patients with social anxiety disorder, 50% for patients with panic disorder, 48% for patients with posttraumatic stress disorder, and 43% for patients with generalized anxiety disorder.

But this isn't just true of depression and anxiety disorders; co-occurrence of psychiatric diagnoses is very common. Decades of research has shown that if you have one diagnosis the likelihood of having another is quite high (e.g., Kessler, Avenevoli et al., 2012; Kessler, Chiu et al., 2005; Plana-Ripoll et al., 2019). This brings into question the distinction between diagnostic categories, and, therefore, the results of treatment studies. If the diagnostic categories aren't reliable then how do I know I'm treating the symptoms that I am said to be treating? And if I'm not really treating what I think I'm treating, then how do I know if it's effective?

The evidence seems to suggest that the DSM isn't delivering on its goals. Even after years of research, the reliability of the diagnostic categories of the DSM isn't great – neither are the treatment outcomes. Though the DSM diagnostic categories are still the standard – at least in the United States – it seems as though they are setting a low bar.

New Models of Classification

Because of the issues with the DSM classification of psychiatric disorders, many have begun developing what they hope to be better classification schemes. While there are many (for an overview see Hayes & Hofmann, 2020), I want to focus my attention on the model proposed by the National Institute of Mental Health (NIMH). Their model is known as RDoC – which stands for Research Domain Criteria.

RDoC was created to address the problems of the DSM categorization. As Uma Vaidyanathan and her colleagues wrote in 2020:

> Contemporary research has identified a variety of problems with the current diagnostic systems. . . . The current dominant model of mental disorders conceptualizes these phenomena as categorical conditions reflecting a simple binary distinction between "well" and "sick." . . . Further, it is increasingly recognized that the current disorder categories represent broad and heterogeneous syndromes rather than specific disease entities.

The developers of the RDoC framework saw the problems with the DSM classification strategy and tried to rectify them.

The avenue they took to rectify the problems of the DSM was to focus on the advances that have occurred in neuroscience research. Vaidyanathan and her colleagues further explained that RDoC allows for mental health issues to be:

> more directly informed by the clinical and translational research that could be more directly informed by the considerable advances in contemporary behavioral neuroscience research. Rather than continuing to focus on psychiatric research endeavors of existing diagnostic classifications, which do not appear to align with patterns of dysfunction in neural circuits, behavior, or genetics, RDoC encourages researchers to instead anchor their hypotheses in the understanding of behavioral, cognitive, and affective neuroscience and to consider how psychiatric symptoms might arise from abnormalities in these symptoms.

The RDoC framework focuses on six domains of human functioning: Negative Valence, Positive Valence, Cognitive Systems, Systems for Social Processes, Arousal/Regulatory Systems, and Sensorimotor Systems. These domains are very complex, so I'll touch just briefly on each domain. But if you want to take a deeper dive, the NIMH has created a website to help walk you through it: www.nimh.nih.gov/research/research-funded-by-nimh/rdoc/constructs/rdoc-matrix.

Negative valence systems include the fear and anxiety system, loss, and what NIMH calls frustrative nonreward – which is the reaction that occurs to the withdrawal or prevention of a reward after sustained effort to get it. Positive valence systems are the reaction that we have when we expect a reward or when we get one, and what we learn from getting these rewards. The cognitive systems refer to our attention, perceptions, language, and memory, and the cognitive control we can exert. Social process systems are about the attachments we form, how we communicate socially, and how we perceive and understand ourselves and others. The arousal and regulatory systems are about how we respond to stimuli in the environment, and also include systems such as our circadian rhythms. Finally, the sensorimotor systems refer to the reflexes, habits, and the agency we have over our motor actions. Each of the domains of RDoC occurs across development and is influenced by the environment we are embedded in.

As the NIMH notes on its website:

> The aim of RDoC is to provide data about basic biological and cognitive processes related to mental health and illness, broadly conceived. New insight generated by research using RDoC framework are intended to inform the development of mental health screening tools, revisions to diagnostic systems, and preventative and treatment interventions.

But how successful have these endeavors been? RDoC has been around for more than a decade now and the evidence is starting to emerge. This early evidence shows promise (Carcone & Ruocco, 2017), but others have begun to point out problems with the framework (Ross & Margolis, 2019). I don't want to spend time detailing all the support and critiques of RDoC, but I would encourage you to look for yourself. I've included some suggested readings at the end of this chapter.

I do want to call attention to what I see as the two major issues with RDoC. The first, RDoC is still a biomedical framework for understanding mental illness. Sure, the frame considers the role of the environment, development, and social processes in mental health, but not systemically. In my reading of RDoC, these things are factors not systems. To return to a quote I presented early in the chapter by George Engel:

> Since systems theory holds that all levels of organization are linked to each other in a hierarchical relationship so that change in one affects change in the others, its adoption as a scientific approach should do much to mitigate the holist-reductionist dichotomy.

To me, the RDoC framework doesn't get far enough away from the holist-reductionist dichotomy. Even though it frames the domains as systems, there isn't much discussion about the interconnectedness of these systems or potential isomorphisms across them. To me, RDoC is looking at factors that are associated with mental illness and mental health, but not rooting itself in systems theory.

Second, RDoC as currently constituted is not useful in psychotherapy. Not to say it couldn't be, but as I read it, the goal of RDoC is to better understand the brain and develop biomedical treatments. Don't get me wrong, I think this type of research is important. I've personally benefited from anti-anxiety medication for nearly a decade. But when I'm sitting with a family whose child is struggling, how will the RDoC framework help me understand what is going on? And how will it help me decide what is important information and what isn't? RDoC does think about psychotherapy, but only about cognitive-behavioral approach – another intervention I would not see as systemic. But by doing that, it limits itself from developing other approaches that may work better.

If you can't tell, I'm not too high on the RDoC framework – at least for what it means for family therapists. I think this approach is so far away from the theoretical grounding of family therapy, that it's likely that family therapists will examine this framework and its resulting diagnoses and again claim "we don't believe in diagnoses." If that happens, I think family therapy would be stuck in the same place it is now.

Family therapists have put forward their own model of diagnosis: relational diagnosis. Relational diagnosis was also developed in response to what was seen as problems with classifications created by psychologists and psychiatrists. As you'll see in the next chapter, relational diagnosis originally had lofty goals, but it hasn't gained the traction that the creators had originally hoped. To me, the issues with relational diagnosis are the same as with the RDoCs – it's not systemic and it's not clinically useful. Before I dive into that, I want to recap the main ideas and arguments in this chapter. I've tried to spell them out plainly so if you need to return to them as you read, you can do so quickly.

Recap: Main Ideas and Arguments

1. **The biomedical model is the dominant model in diagnostic practice.** The biomedical model mainly assumes that mental health disorders occur within an individual. As such, the diagnostic process for mental disorders is focused on identifying symptoms, providing a working diagnosis, and applying individual-focused treatment. If the treatment is unsuccessful, then new information needs to be gathered to provide a better diagnosis and hopefully better treatment. This model is the most widely used and currently the only one that receives reimbursement from insurance companies.

2. **The current iteration of the DSM, DSM 5, is rooted in the bio-medical model.** The goal or rooting of DSM 5 in the biomedical model was to create valid and reliable diagnostic categories that would allow for effective intervention. Research has suggested that the promises of the DSM to provide this have fallen short.

3. **New diagnostic frameworks, such as RDoC, have been put forward to improve upon the DSM.** While these models have the potential to provide better diagnostic categories, they also fall short. Specifically, they are still rooted in the biomedical model, and still assume that mental disorders reside mainly within an individual. What's more, these models aren't very useful in psychotherapy. Because they are based on a biomedical model, they don't provide a theoretical explanation that can help a therapist understand how or why the issue is occurring.

4. **For a diagnosis to be useful in psychotherapy it needs to be built on a valid and clinically useful theory.** If a diagnosis is not based on a clinically valid theory, then it can do little to inform a therapist as to how they should intervene.

Chapter 2

Relational Diagnosis

When I began my master's degree in family therapy in 2007, there was one book that I was the most excited to read. It was called the *Handbook of Relational Diagnosis and Dysfunctional Family Patterns*. I had high hopes for this book. As a novice therapist, I was hoping that this book would be the guide I needed to decode what was really happening in families. I was hoping that by reading this book, I would be able to unlock the secret of how to be a family therapist and how to do family therapy. I hoped it would help me see families and their problems in a whole new way.

But that book really let me down. What I hoped would be a theoretically-driven, process-oriented model of conceptualizing family problems, ended up being the opposite. I found the book to be more like the DSM than to the ideas of Bowen, Minuchin, Satir, and White that I was reading. In some cases, the book gave me a set of symptoms that I could look for, but it didn't help me understand why these symptoms were present or what kept them going. Unlike many of the other books I read, I didn't find myself returning to the *Handbook of Relational Diagnosis* again and again. It just sat on my shelf gathering dust.

What this book turned out to be is very different from the goals that those who created it espoused. So, I want to start this chapter by tracing the history of relational diagnosis. I'll then provide an example of how a relational diagnosis could be made. Finally, I'll argue that while this line of work is important especially to family therapists' ability to diagnose, it can't be the only diagnostic method we pursue.

The History of Relational Diagnosis

The concept of relational diagnosis has a long history in family therapy. Family systems thinkers tried, with little success, to influence revisions to the DSM-III in the late '70s. When DSM-IV was being developed, family therapists again wanted to push for the inclusion of relational diagnosis. To this end, a Task Force on Family Diagnosis and Classification was

DOI: 10.4324/9781003295907-3

created in 1987. This organization met with other organizations focusing on family diagnosis – the Group for the Advancement of Psychiatry's Task Force on the Family and the American Association for Marriage and Family Therapy (AAFMT) – in 1988.

Wayne Denton, a representative of AAMFT, was tasked with drafting a mission statement for these working groups. In consultation with others from these groups, this mission statement was published in 1989. The mission statement began by squarely rooting relational diagnosis in systems theory. It says:

> Although there are different approaches to family therapy, a common thread is an acknowledgement of the influence of general systems theory. Whereas in traditional psychopathology, the interest is in what symptoms tell us about the inner workings of the individual, in family systems approaches the interest is in what symptoms tell us about the interactions among family members. . . . Defining the scope of the DSM as including only disorders representing the dysfunction within the individual constitutes a subtle, and probably unplanned, theoretical assumption which has great significance for family therapists. It excludes problems that emerge from disturbed relational patterns and symptoms.
>
> (Denton & Coalition, 1989)

Denton is making explicit the task force's theoretical grounding – general systems theory – and is arguing for a model of diagnosis rooted in this theory.

Denton expands on this argument in greater detail in his chapter from the *Handbook of Relational Diagnosis*. In that chapter, he writes about the medical model and then discusses George Engel's biopsychosocial model and general systems theory, writing:

> The biopsychosocial model conceptualizes nature as arranged on a hierarchical continuum ranging from molecules, through individuals, to families, to societies. While each system level interacts with those levels above and below it, each level also represents a 'dynamic whole' in its own right.
>
> A logical extension of this idea would be that each system level can have its own type of dysfunction. General systems theory (and the biopsychosocial model) maintains that dysfunction in one system will impact the other system levels. However, for that impact to produce exactly the same result in every case would require that every system level have no heterogeneity. For example, suppose that an individual experiences a double bind in family communication. What the double-bind hypothesis failed to recognize is that there is more

to a family than simply the fact that the members may convey double binds. Each family will have a host of strengths and weaknesses, which will in some ways distinguish it from other families that also might communicate in double binds. This hypothesis also ignored the fact that the individual on the receiving end of the double-bind message will have had a variety of learning experiences and a unique genetic makeup. Further, that individual will live in a specific community and culture that will be different from the ones in which other individuals who might experience communicational double binds reside. Thus, while coping with double-bind communication might be difficult and undesirable, it seems reasonable to assume that this type of interaction will affect different individuals differently and that all symptomatology has multiple causes rather than only one.

Again, Denton is arguing that understanding symptoms requires examining multiple systems and the linkages between those systems. He is squarely setting the relational diagnosis on the path of being systemic.

But the goal of this working group didn't pan out. Florence Kaslow, the editor of the *Handbook of Relational Diagnosis*, described how tension and friction in the working group led to problems. In the first chapter of her book, she writes:

> The Coalition met two to four times a year [beginning in] 1988. . . . Many meetings were devoted to generating a list of diagnoses that might accurately describe various prevalent marital and family dysfunctional patterns. Delineating these dysfunctional interactive patterns and finding descriptive terminology for these patterns that could elicit widespread agreement among participants proved extremely difficult.

Though Denton and Kaslow's goal was to ground relational diagnosis in systems theory, it seems like others in the group weren't on board. I wasn't in those meetings, but it seems that the goal may have gotten lost when trying to get widespread agreement.

Despite the disagreements, the Coalition continued. Kaslow was eventually contacted by a publishing company, drew upon the expertise of some of the members of the Coalition, and wrote the *Handbook of Relational Diagnosis*. It was published in 1996. At the end of the book, Kaslow articulates what she hopes to see as the next steps for relational diagnosis. She writes:

> soon after this volume is published and we start to receive constructive input from our readers, we hope to begin work on Volume II – perhaps a manual of relation disorders – to offer a

language that has achieved high consensus in categories that will be delineated in a more uniform manner, so that more meaningful dialogues can occur among and between therapists, their patients, and those of significance in the larger ecosystem. The schema that has begun to emerge will be validated, expanded, and refined and will enable therapists and researchers in the international family of family therapists and researchers finally to have a nosology of family diagnosis that is applicable across geographical and cultural boundaries.

The second volume was never published.

But Kaslow and others again pushed for relational diagnosis in 2006. That year in a special section of the *Journal of Family Psychology*, she and other researchers made the argument for relational diagnosis with the hope of influencing the writing of DSM-5. Throughout this special section, strong arguments are made as to why the DSM needs relational diagnosis. But one of the last articles in this section spells out the reasons why it has been so hard to make headway. Jay Lebow and Kristina Coop Gordon write:

> First, there has been a lack of consensus about exactly what relational assessment and diagnosis entail. . . . Numerous rich and valuable ideas for dimensions of assessment and relational categories have been described, but even within a particular view of how to assess relational dimensions, there has been no consensus about which of these dimension or categories were most worthy of attention. . . .
>
> A second constraint is the unavoidable presence of complexity in any effort at relational assessment. Even within particular orientations of viewing problems, few definitive well-accepted, evidence-based operational definitions of difficulties have emerged. . . .
>
> A third, related constraint has been that empirical testing of how to best assess relational understandings has lagged behind the development of elegant theories describing family systems. . . .
>
> A final, closely related obstacle to adopting relational diagnosis, and perhaps the most potent, involves the political process that is part of the evolution of diagnostic system. The DSM, with its various inconsistencies and curiosities, speaks to an underlying process that is highly political.

If you look at DSM-5, you'll see that Lebow and Coop Gordon were right. Relationships and relationship processes seem an afterthought in the DSM-5. Whether it's political, or just the complexity of relational assessment, relational diagnosis in 2006 was still not codified.

A more recent push to develop relational diagnosis occurred in 2016. In a special issue of the journal *Family Process*, it was argued that relational diagnosis was an idea whose "time had come." Jay Lebow (2015), the editor of *Family Process* at the time, began the issue by saying:

> This issue offers one of the most important collections of articles ever published by *Family Process*: a special section devoted to relational diagnosis. This section does not in any sense represent the birth of a new concept. . . . Yet [previous] efforts were preliminary, a precursor to the more detailed scientific study of relational diagnosis. The special section in this issue edited by Marianne Wamboldt demonstrates the remarkable maturation of this body of work over the last two decades.

When I came across these articles, I had a similar feeling to what I felt when I originally came across the *Handbook of Relational Diagnosis*. Again, I thought I would finally be able to read a systemically grounded, clinically useful diagnostic process that I could use in my practice and with my students. But again, I was let down.

Don't get me wrong, I think that these articles represented a big step for relational diagnosis. The research summarized within the issue represents 41 field studies that have occurred across the globe. This research was rigorous and important. It was just a step toward the medical model and a step away from systems theory and biopsychosocial approaches. Let me show you what I mean.

In one article, Marianne Wamboldt, Anthony Cordaro Jr., and Diana Clarke (2015) proposed the relational diagnosis of "Parent-Child Relational Problem (PCRP)." This diagnosis had two criteria. To meet diagnostic classification the parent-child dyad needed one symptom from the first criterion and two symptoms from the second criterion. These criteria and symptoms include:

Criterion 1 – Relationship dissatisfaction or distress occurs more days than not during the past month as evidenced by at least one of the following: pervasive sense of unhappiness with relationship (parent or child); thoughts of running away that are more than transitory (child); thoughts of relinquishing care of the child that are more than transitory (parent); perceived need (parent, child, or clinician) of professional help for the relationships.

Criterion 2 – Significant impact of relational dissatisfaction on behavioral, cognitive, or affective systems, as evidenced by at least two of the following for either the caregiver or child: conflict resolution difficulties; overinvolvement; underinvolvement; pervasive pattern of negative attributions regarding the other's intentions; and/ or interactions with or thoughts about the others are frequently marked by intense and persistent levels of any of the following – anger, apathy, or sadness.

To test whether this relational diagnosis was valid, the researchers recruited 133 parent-child dyads. The average age of the children recruited was 11 years old and more than half of the children were male (57.9%). The caregivers were mostly mothers (85.7%). The researcher assessed the dyads in multiple ways and asked the clinicians assessing the dyad if they thought the diagnosis was clinically useful.

In summarizing their results, Wamboldt, Cordaro Jr., and Clarke wrote:

> The main findings from this study indicate that clinicians can reliably diagnose PCRP in a clinical population of child-parent dyads given the use of clinical information including the parent/caregiver narrative of the child-parent relationship and child report of parental bonding and perceived criticism to and from the parent/caregiver. . . . Our intention was to develop and test a definition with reliable criteria, such that it could be widely used in clinical settings as well as epidemiological clinical research settings.
>
> While the definition we proposed will clearly need to be refined, it did achieve good test-retest reliability (interclass kappa of .58) . . . which indicates that clinicians of a variety of training background, years of experiences, and theoretical bents can agree on whether these constructs are present or not.

Do you remember our discussion of kappa from Chapter 1? This statistic describes the likelihood that if two clinicians interviewed the same person and made the same diagnosis, this was not due to chance. Remember too, that Allen Frances, the head of the DSM-IV taskforce suggested that a kappa above .6 was acceptable, but still not great. In other words, it may be that some of the same issues we find in the diagnoses of the DSM might be finding their way into relational diagnosis.

Regardless of the kappa values, the work of developing reliable classifications of relational disorders is still ongoing. It may be that in the coming decades the vision of Florence Kaslow will be realized, and we will have a manual like the DSM that contains relation diagnostic categories. If that does happen, I think the field of family therapy could benefit greatly. But not in the way I'm advocating for in this book. I don't think the current process of relational diagnosis has the same goal that it originally set out with. In my reading, systems theory is all but ignored; little attention is paid to systems and their role in mental health. And I don't think researchers or clinicians are studying relational diagnosis with the goal of creating a therapeutically useful form of assessment to guide treatment. To me, relational diagnosis isn't the biopsychosocial framework that Engel and Woods advocated for, it's the distillation of the biomedical model to relationships.

However, I do think that the current goal of relational diagnosis is a good one. In my reading of the current relational diagnosis thinkers, the purpose of creating diagnostic categories centers in one main area: insurance reimbursement. As someone who makes part of their living from insurance reimbursement, I think this is an important goal. If family therapists can't get paid for their work, we won't be around for long. But if this is the only goal of relational diagnosis, I don't think it will be clinically useful as the originators hoped.

Example of Relational Diagnosis

Before I explain more about why I think relational diagnosis isn't clinically useful, I want to show you how I think relational diagnosis would look in practice. I wasn't trained in relational diagnosis the same way I was trained in diagnosis based on the DSM; nor are there a lot of examples out there of how this happens outside of research studies. But I still want to present a hypothetical case example of making a relational diagnosis. I hope that this thought exercise illuminates the process of relational diagnosis but also shows its limitations.

Let's meet Candice and her 15-year-old-daughter Lindsey. They are going to get the diagnosis of parent-child relational problem. I'd advise you to check out the diagnostic criteria again. I'm going to assume that Candice and Lindsey completed paperwork that indicated to me that they were arguing frequently and had trouble communicating.

Therapist: Candice and Lindsey, it's nice to meet you both and thanks for coming in. I'm going to start off today by asking you a few questions to get a better understanding of what's been going on between you two. If I ask you a question that you don't feel comfortable answering, just let me know. Does that sound ok?

Candice: Yes, that fine.

Lindsey: <is staring at her phone not looking up>

Therapist: Candice, can I start with you? In my paperwork it says that you and Lindsey have been fighting and having trouble communicating. Can you tell me more about that?

Candice: Sure. It's been really bad I'd say for the past few months. Lindsey won't listen, she's always staring at her phone. If I try and take it away, she gets really angry. She's started failing her classes. She says she's not on drugs or anything, but I'm not sure. Basically, I've done everything I can and I'm just exhausted.

Therapist: It sounds like things have been really hard lately. Do you see it the same, Lindsey?

Lindsey: Sure.

Candice: Get off your phone, Lindsey. God, can you pay attention for one second?

Lindsey: <rolls eyes>

Candice: <grabs Lindsey's phone> Answer the question.

Lindsey: Fuck you, mom, give me my phone.

Candice: No. You need to pay attention and answer the question.

Lindsey: Fine, my mom's a bitch.

Candice: Watch it. We are not going to do this right now.

Therapist: Why don't we slow down a bit? Would it be better if I just talked with you first, Candice? Lindsey, can I walk you to the waiting room and you can hang out there for a bit?

Lindsey: I want my phone.

Candice: Fine, take it.

Therapist: Thanks for talking with me, Candice.

Candice: I'm so sorry about her. She's just so exhausting.

Therapist: It sounds like the two of you have not been doing well, tell me a bit more.

Candice: Well, like I said, it started a few months ago. She just started getting really nasty and angry. Calling me names, cursing, and not doing anything I tell her.

Therapist: Ok. So, this has been going on for a few months? How is it different than before?

Candice: Well, I mean, we've always had fights, but since she started high school, things have been going downhill fast. I think it's because we got her a phone. Since she's gotten it, our fights have gotten worse and worse.

Therapist: And these fights, what typically happens? Does it feel like the same thing over and over again, or is it different each time?

Candice: I don't know. It feels the same. Like yesterday, I was talking to her about cleaning her room and she was on her phone not paying attention. Just like now, I grabbed her phone. She started yelling, so I started yelling. We go at it for a while until she slams her bedroom door.

Therapist: So what I just saw when we first started is pretty typical?

Candice: Yeah. She doesn't listen so I take her phone and then we just yell.

Therapist: And how often does this happen? Like every day? A couple times a week?

Candice: It's basically every day. I mean we don't have a blowup every day, but there hasn't been a day I can think of where we haven't yelled at each other recently.

Therapist: Ok, and has it ever gotten worse than this? Like is slamming the door typically how Lindsey responds? Or are there other things too?

Candice: I mean, door slamming is typical, but she's run away a few times, snuck out a few times. Sometimes I'll go knock on her door after we fight and she's not there. It used to scare me but now I'm just over it.

Therapist: Over it? How so?

Candice: I've tried everything. I've cried, I've yelled, I've tried to ground her. Take away her phone. I just don't know what to do any more. And some days I just want to give up and let her do whatever she wants.

Therapist: It does sound exhausting and disheartening. You mentioned that you think it started with the phone or when she started high school?

Candice: Yeah. We got her the phone when she started high school.

Therapist: Gotcha. So you think this is what caused the shift?

Candice: I guess. I think maybe originally but now even if she doesn't have her phone she's still like this.

Therapist: Like what?

Candice: Angry, flippant, doesn't listen. I'm starting to think it's just who she is.

Therapist: Okay. And is this behavior just with you or does it happen elsewhere?

Candice: I mean you'd think she's two different people. At school she's fine. Her grades are good, her teachers like her, she does well. But when she walks through the door, she turns.

Therapist: There's a disconnect between who she is at home and who she is at school?

Candice: Big time.

Therapist: Ok. And her teachers aren't concerned about her?

Candice: Nope. They love her. They say she's great. It kinda pisses me off when I talk to them. I want that girl, but I'm left with all the shit.

Therapist: And does Lindsey ever seem depressed? Or stressed? Or anxious?

Candice: If she does, she hides it well. I talked to our doctor about it, and she didn't seem to think she was depressed or anything, that's why she sent us to you.

Therapist: Ok. I want to make sure I'm getting this right. Lindsey does well in school, hasn't been diagnosed with any mental health conditions, and seems to be well liked by her teachers and peers?

Candice: Yes. That's correct.

Therapist: But since she started high school and got a phone her behavior at home has changed.

Candice: Yes, changed a lot.

Therapist: You and Lindsey fight most days? And they typically involve yelling and slamming doors?

Candice: Yes.

Therapist: And Lindsey has run away and snuck out a few times during the past few months as well?

Candice: Right.

Therapist: And where does she go?

Candice: The first time I found her at her friend's house. She told her friend's mom all sorts of thing about me and how bad I was.

Therapist: Like what?

Candice: Basically, she said I was a controlling bitch. That I don't listen to her and that I don't really care about her or love her.

Therapist: And how did you react when you heard she said those things?

Candice: The first time it really hurt. I cried a lot. But now, it's just what happens. I mean, last time she ran away, I didn't even look for her. I figured she'd come back eventually and trying to find her and bring her back would just make it worse.

Therapist: Ok. And when things get really heated, have there ever been any hitting or pushing or anything like that?

Candice: I mean I've wanted to, but I'd never do it. That's part of the reason I just disconnect now. If I keep escalating who knows where it would go. And at this point I feel like whatever I do isn't going to work anyway.

Therapist: Alright. And these fights with Lindsey, anything else you'd want me to know? I want to spend time talking to her as well, I just want to make sure I've got the information you wanted to share.

Candice: No, not really. I just want it fixed. I just need Lindsey to stop.

Therapist: Ok, I want to talk with Lindsey for a bit. Come with me, and I'll take you to the waiting room.

I'm not going to provide a hypothetical conversation with Lindsey. But let's assume that she has a different take on the situation but confirms what her mom says in terms of the symptoms of a parent-child relation problem. If that's the case, then it seems they would meet the diagnostic criteria I summarized earlier. They have a pervasive sense of unhappiness about the relationship; Lindsey has run away; there is marked escalation of behavior and affect; there is strong negative attributions about behavior, and positive interactions are explained away; and finally, Candice is showing anger and apathy.

The Problems With Relational Diagnosis

For me, I think this type of interview could be important. If parent-child relational problem was a codified diagnosis, and I would be able to use it for insurance reimbursement, then I think that all family therapists and their clients would benefit from this type of interview. If the end goal of relational diagnosis is that it gets people access to care that they need, then relational diagnosis as presently constituted is a worthwhile goal. Many have made the case that treating relational issues and having relational diagnosis could potentially prevent the onset or exacerbation of mental illness, and would save insurers money in the long run (e.g., Clawson et al., 2018; Negash et al., 2022). In my mind there is a strong case to be made for being able to provide services and get reimbursed from a relational diagnosis.

However, getting reimbursed by insurance and having a clinically relevant diagnosis are two separate things. If you look at the example I provided, you can tell that Candice and Lindsey have a parent-child relational problem – but not much else. We know little about the larger family system; we don't know anything about the family's culture or identities; we don't know the processes or interactions that created or maintain this problem; we don't know if this conflict is a symptom that the system needs; we don't know if it's a feature of the system or just a bug.

If we knew all these things, it would be much easier to decide on a course of treatment. If the real problem lies in the fact that Candice's partner had an affair and that she discovered it the same time that Lindsey started high school, treating the parent-child problem may not help. It may be that Lindsey came out to her mom as non-binary and her mom dismissed or punished her for that. It may be that there is another child in the home who struggles with health problems and this stress has strained Candice and Lindsey's relationship.

If we only know the problem exists but don't know why it exists or how it developed, our therapy is going to be less effective. We may try to fix the problem by making Lindsey resilient to a toxic system, or we may miss important context that may invalidate Candice and make her disown parts of herself to be the parent the therapist tells her she "should be." We may apply a model of therapy that has been shown effective in treating parent-child problems, and never realize that the problem stabilizes the system. If we fix the problem, we may destabilize the system.

To me the main problem with relational diagnosis in its current form is that it looks more like the biomedical model than a biopsychosocial model; it looks more like the DSM than the work of Haley, Bowen, Minuchin, or Satir. To me, relational diagnosis isn't systemic. Though Denton and Kaslow had hopes that it might be, it's just become a list of symptoms that don't explain much.

But I think there can be a better way. A way that coincides with the work of relational diagnosis but makes it more clinically useful. I think family systems theory can be used to help us create diagnoses that are clinically meaningful, help explain how and why, and provide a context of understanding that can guide treatment. I think that if family therapists can learn to create accurate systemic diagnoses, they can intervene more effectively for their clients. But before we dive into that, I think it's important that we are clear on the main points of this chapter. Like in Chapter 1, I've tried to summarize this argument clearly, so you can revisit them as you read.

Recap: Main Ideas and Arguments

1. Family therapists have for decades been critical of the biomedical roots of diagnosis – and the DSM. Over the years there have been efforts to put forth models that could complement or compete with the diagnostic criteria of the DSM. However, these models have typically fallen short. One example of this is relational diagnosis.

2. Relational diagnosis was originally designed to be built on family systems theory. Through the efforts of Florence Kaslow and others, the *Handbook of Relational Diagnosis and Dysfunctional Family Patterns* was completed in 1996. This volume outlined the goals of relational diagnosis and gave examples of possible diagnostic categories. Kaslow took up the effort again in 2006, and the journal *Family Process* again pushed for relational diagnosis in 2016. Now, it seems that the goal of relational diagnosis is to allow family therapists to get reimbursed by insurance. While this is an important goal, in doing so, relational diagnosis has lost its grounding in family systems theory.

3. By losing its grounding in family systems theory, the clinical utility of relational diagnosis has greatly diminished. Relational diagnosis, as currently constituted, provides little guidance for couple and family therapists. While it may help family therapists receive insurance reimbursement in the future; it does very little to advance systemic interventions.

Part II

Family Systems Theory and Systemic Diagnosis

Before I jump in and make the case for systemic diagnosis, I need to be transparent – I'm biased. I like to think that this bias is an informed biased, but it's a bias nonetheless.

In my job, I've supervised and worked with psychiatrists, psychologists, social workers, mental health counsellors, and family therapists. I've also spent much of my career thinking about mental health disorders and relational and social systems. I researched and studied these ideas and argued that family systems theory needs to be the grounding idea of psychotherapy practice. In this part of the book, I'm going to try and convince you that systemic diagnosis, rooted in family systems theory, is the model of diagnosis that can lead to the best possible treatment of the individuals, couples, and families we work with.

But don't just take my word for it.

There are limitations and problems with systemic diagnosis. In Part II of this book, I'm going to talk about some of them and offer what I see as potential avenues of study and practice to overcome these limitations. Yet, if you want to diagnose well, especially using the systemic model, you need to be skeptical of my argument. Whether you are training to become a therapist or if you've been practicing for years, just accepting and applying the model of systemic diagnosis won't help you provide better care for your clients. You need to challenge and critique these ideas. I know that's a lot to ask. If you are training to become a therapist, you are already getting a lot of information thrown at you. If you are currently practicing, there often isn't space to add any additional work to your busy schedule. However, I think that good therapists, who want to provide good therapy, need to take time to wrestle with new ideas. So, as you read, I'd encourage you not to take what I say at face value. Rather, bring your knowledge, experience, and expertise, and see if what I'm arguing holds up.

With that made clear, I want to set the stage to try and make a compelling argument for systemic diagnosis. To make it, we need to be clear about a few terms: theory, diagnosis, and intervention. And that's where

DOI: 10.4324/9781003295907-4

we start out. In Chapter 3, I'm going to talk about what I see as a bad trend in family therapy – lumping theory, diagnosis, and intervention into one entity. I'll argue that lumping them together has gotten the field of family therapy stuck. To get us unstuck we need to see theory, diagnosis, and intervention as three distinct but connected components of good therapy. I'll explore all of this in Chapter 3 and argue that if we understand the distinction between theory, diagnosis, and intervention, we can do all of them better.

Chapter 4 is all about family systems theory. I'll present the assumptions that family systems theory is built on, and the hypotheses of family systems theory that extend from these assumptions. Specifically, I propose that family systems theory has two main hypotheses – the family is an autonomous system, and the family is an adaptable system. I'll explain what these terms mean and how these two hypotheses predict and explain family interactions. In Chapter 5, I'll revisit the connection between theory and diagnosis and demonstrate how family systems theory can be used to gather the information you'll need to make systemic diagnoses.

Chapter 6 is all about taking the information and using it to make a systemic diagnosis. Unlike other models of diagnosis, systemic diagnosis doesn't have predetermined categories of systems. It assumes that systems are all going to develop interactions and patterns based on the unique developmental context that a family experiences. Chapter 6 doesn't contain diagnostic criteria or symptoms of good and bad families, or even unique family types. But it does contain a way to categorize the history, structure, and boundaries of a system. What's more, in Chapter 6 we'll discuss how to use a systemic diagnosis as a roadmap of intervention. I will show you how to take your systemic diagnosis and find intervention points to move systems from disintegrating to thriving trajectories.

Chapter 7 is all about the problems and the potential of systemic diagnosis. To me, understanding the limitations and problems with any theory or diagnostic model is fundamental to doing it well. In Chapter 7, I'll present what I see as the largest problems with systemic diagnosis, and I will talk about ways I think these problems can be overcome through research and clinical work. I'm also going to discuss the benefits of systemic diagnosis and how it could transform the work we do with clients.

Chapter 3

The Trinity

Theory, Diagnosis, and Intervention

I grew up Mormon. Though I haven't practiced for most of my adult life, there are many theological questions I remember talking about when I was younger. One of the earliest happened with my dad. When I was in my teens in 1990s, there always seemed to be a question swirling around Mormonism: Are Mormons Christian? I remember bringing this up to my dad and asking him why this question existed. My thought was, "Mormons believe in Jesus, so that makes them Christian, right?" My dad, who studies not just Mormonism but all religions, was happy to respond.

Now, you might be thinking, "What does any of this have to do with theory, diagnosis, and research?" But just hang on a bit, and I'll try to answer that question.

What I thought was a simple question about whether Mormons were Christian or not, turned out to be a conversation with my dad that wandered through early Christianity, the Nicene Creed, reformers like Martin Luther, Mormonism's founder Joseph Smith, and even a small tangent into Zoroastrianism. To be honest, I don't remember all the particulars, but my oversimplified memory is that the reason it was often argued that Mormons aren't believed to be Christian is that they view the Trinity – God, Jesus, and the Holy Spirit – different than most Christian denominations.

Again, this is an oversimplification, but most Christians believe that God, Jesus, and the Holy Spirit are one God – in many cases the word consubstantial is used to describe this; while Mormons believe that God, Jesus, and the Holy Spirit are three physically separate beings. In other words, because Mormons view the Trinity differently than most Christians, the argument arises that maybe Mormons aren't Christians.

I'm not going to weigh in on who has it right – I'm agnostic when it comes to most theological questions. But I do like a good argument, so even as a nonbeliever it has been interesting over the years to look at arguments put forth by both camps about why they believe what they believe, and the evidence that they use to support their claims. When new ideas get juxtaposed with old ideas, I think it helps these ideas become heightened and better clarified.

DOI: 10.4324/9781003295907-5

In family therapy, we also have a trinity – theory, diagnosis, and intervention. These are the things that family therapists learn and do. But most family therapists and family therapy researchers see them as the same thing. If you look at most family therapy textbooks, they conflate the idea of theory and intervention. Many of the models of intervention are described in textbooks as "Family Therapy Theories." And most see diagnosis as part of the theory/model. For example, Structural Family Therapy is at once a theory, a way to diagnose, and a model of intervention. The same could be said for Bowen's approach or Strategic Family Therapy.

I'm not sure if a group of family therapists got together to make a declaration that theory, diagnosis, and intervention are consubstantial. If they did, I didn't get the invite. But in my experience, this is the mainstream belief of family therapy. In fact, I think this assumption is what underlies the idea that family therapists "don't believe in diagnosis." If theory, diagnosis, and intervention are all the same, then we can easily discard one of them, because if we can do one, we can do them all.

I find this approach problematic. When we conflate theory, diagnosis, and intervention, we obscure the purpose of each. This ends up reducing the effectiveness of our practice, and our ability to innovate. I find that family therapists are trained almost exclusively in intervention. Students may have a class on diagnosis, but that course typically covers the DSM. Students may learn about theory, but when you ask them to describe theory, they talk about intervention. Lumping together theory, diagnosis, and intervention, in my estimation, has pushed the field of family therapy toward only teaching, researching, and applying interventions. Intervention is flashy. That's what therapists want to learn and what our clients want us to do. It's what gets grant funding to show that family therapy can help people with mental health problems. But intervention is less effective without good theory and diagnosis. If we assume they are the same, we don't study, teach, or use them as they are intended.

I'm not purporting to be Martin Luther or Joseph Smith, but I do think family therapy needs to reform our understanding of the trinity. Are theory, diagnosis, and intervention connected? Yes, but they are not the same. Each has a distinct purpose.

Theory in Family Therapy

What is theory? And what is the purpose of theory in family therapy?

Let's answer the first question first. I like the definition given by Katherine Allen and Angela Henderson (2016). In their book, *Family Theories*, they define theory as:

> a strategy to describe, interpret, and/or explain a phenomenon. . . .
> A theory, then, offers us a compelling storyline that helps us interpret the
> how and why of a situation or experience where we need to know why.

Theories help us describe or explain something. They give us a way of interpreting or understanding the "why" or "how" of something.

Throughout human history one of the biggest phenomena humans have tried to understand is their own existence. Lutherans, Mormons, and Zoroastrians all have their own theories. Religion, in part, was developed by someone who said – I can explain why we are here. Scientists have sought to explain this as well. If you haven't noticed, religion and science don't always agree. Both have theories that interpret and explain the question, "Why are we here?" but the evidence used to support that claim is very different.

Part of the reason for this is that religion and science rest on different epistemologies. Epistemology is the study of knowledge. It examines how we know what we know or how we justify what we know. We can "know" things in lots of different ways. Your epistemology helps you prioritize a type of knowing or a type of evidence to support what you know. Knowing something in a religious context is different than knowing something in a scientific context. Religion and science have different epistemologies which means that the evidence they use to justify their knowledge has resulted in different theories to explain the same phenomena.

This will be a bit reductive, but to illustrate this point let's assume that science uses the theory of evolution to explain human existence while religion uses the theory of God. The theory of evolution posits that humans exist because of natural selection. The theory of God posits that humans exist because God created them. Which one is right? That depends on what you think constitutes evidence to justify knowledge. It depends on your epistemology.

Theories are all built on epistemologies. To justify a claim, you must decide beforehand what type of evidence can justify it. Currently, family therapy is mostly taught in academic institutions. The knowledge created in academic institutions is historically and currently rooted mainly in what is known as a positivist epistemology. This epistemology holds that we can discover the truth of a phenomena through empirical evidence gained through the scientific method. This epistemology assumes that scientific fact or consensus is reached when we have the preponderance of evidence that supports a claim.

But positive epistemology isn't the only way family therapy is taught. We also rely on expertise gained through experience. Not every issue that is presented in family therapy has been scientifically studied – nor can it be. That is why family therapists need experience and supervision. We can gain expertise through experience. We tend to get better at things that we've done over and over again and we can also gain expertise by receiving supervision from someone who is more experienced (Hill et al., 2017). They pass on their knowledge gained through experience so that novice family therapists don't have to relearn everything through trial and error. Experienced therapists train the next generation of therapists through mentorship, oversight, and passing on knowledge. If you've ever been to a family therapy conference, sometimes a person will present a description or explanation of a phenomena related to the family relying on clinical anecdotes or videos. The way they justify their knowledge or theory is through experience. They may have decades working with families and this experience has given them insight that scientific research couldn't find.

To me good family therapy theory rests on a positivist and an experienced-based epistemology. We can justify our theories and our knowledge through research and experience. We can validate our explanations and descriptions through the results of longitudinal or experimental research, but also through doing the work of family therapy. Too often, however, we prioritize one over the other. This can be seen when family therapy anoints a new guru. Often these gurus have lots of experience but don't have the research to back up their claims. On the other hand, a data-only approach to family therapy also falls short. Any data we collect through research to try and support a theory are going to be flawed. We should also be wary of those who only rely on research to justify what they are doing.

So, to return to the first question I posed, "What is theory?" I want to alter my original answer just a bit. Theory in family therapy is a strategy used to describe, explain, or interpret a phenomenon through research and experience.

Now let's answer the second question, "What is the purpose of theory in family therapy?"

To answer this second question, we need to talk about another factor on which theory rests: assumptions. An assumption is what we believe to be true. It is the starting point for theory. The purpose of theory in family therapy is rooted in its assumption. To me this assumption is rooted in a story told to me by one of my supervisors, Jerry.

In one of our earliest supervision meetings, Jerry described to me and the other students his journey into family therapy. He'd been trained as a social worker at the University of Chicago and upon graduating began working with kids with emotional issues. Jerry quickly became frustrated with his ability to help these kids. He could get them to do better in the therapy room, but once they got home the same problem would happen again. When he tried to bring the parents into the therapy room, he had no idea how to navigate what was going on in front of him. Frustrated with his training, he found family therapy and found better tools to work with kids and families.

This story isn't novel. In fact, it's probably how lots of people came to family therapy before it was developed as a degree program that universities granted. The assumption of traditional psychotherapy was that problems existed within the individual; family therapy pushed back against that assumption.

In pushing back on the original psychotherapy assumption, family therapists based their theories on different assumptions. Family therapy theories assume that the family is the context where human flourishing and suffering occurs. These theories assume that the family constitutes an entity that is distinct from other human-relationship entities. Because of its distinctness, families are the unit of intervention that must be addressed to alleviate issues and problems.

But are these assumptions valid? Are families really the important context for human suffering and flourishing? Are family relationships really distinct from other relationships? Is the family really where we should intervene? To validate these assumptions, theorists create propositions or hypotheses to test these assumptions. Depending on the epistemology, theorists devise ways to test or gather evidence to support these propositions. If they can accumulate enough evidence, they may claim that the hypotheses of their theory are valid. And if the hypotheses are valid, then the assumptions on which their theory rest must also be valid. If the evidence doesn't support their propositions, then they need to change their assumptions and rework their hypotheses.

It's not uncommon for theorists working with the same assumptions to have different theories, hypotheses, or means of gathering evidence. In fact, that is good for growing knowledge. Though different theories have the same assumptions, they may distill these down into propositions that test very different things. When this is done, it allows for debate. Debate often helps to clarify and heighten ideas that are similar but different in meaningful ways.

In family therapy, there are many different theories that explain, describe, and interpret family relationships. But they all rest on many of the same assumptions. They all assume that the quality of our closest relationships determines that quality of our lives. To improve people's lives and their mental health, we can't ignore the context of their relationships. These assumptions are what give rise to the purpose of theory in family therapy. Family therapy theories create better knowledge and understanding about family relationships. The better we understand human family relationships, the better we can diagnosis and intervene. As we do this better, we improve human flourishing and reduce suffering.

Theory, however, doesn't tell us how to intervene with clients. Rather it tells us what is important and what is not in family relationships. It allows us a storyline to describe and explain the myriad of experiences families bring to therapy. No family's experience is the same, but theory gives us a roadmap on how interpret to family dynamic. Theory gives us the way to make accurate diagnoses.

Diagnosis in Family Therapy

What Is Diagnosis? And What Is the Purpose of Diagnosis in Family Therapy?

If you remember, in Chapter 1, I talked about the traditional form of diagnosis. Diagnosis was defined as both a "process and classification scheme." In other words, to diagnose you had to go through the process of gathering information and determining if what you gathered fit into the categories of a specific scheme. The traditional form of diagnosis found in the DSM is rooted in biomedical theories. The main assumption of these theories is that mental health problems stem from biological issues in the brain and body. This assumption creates the list of symptoms that reflect the theories.

As I just noted, family therapy theories are built on different assumptions. These are assumptions that were originally part of the push for relational diagnosis. If you remember, in Chapter 2, Wayne Denton wrote about how the classification scheme of relational diagnosis was to be rooted in family systems theory – a theory built on the assumptions described earlier. I argued that relational diagnosis lost its systemic grounding, and in part abandoned the assumptions on which family therapy was originally built.

But, if you return to the examples that I provided in those chapters, you see the connection between theory and diagnosis. In those examples, I asked lots of questions. These questions reflect the assumptions and theory on which each model of diagnosis is built. In Chapter 1, I asked questions which focused on the individual and the individual symptoms. When Dave brought up his mom, it wasn't a path I explored. And theoretically, that makes sense. If I assume that Dave's issue exists within him, then a conversation about his mom and their relationship isn't necessary and may in fact distract me from the important information. In Chapter 2, I asked a bit about individual symptoms, but mostly about the mother-daughter relationship. These questions assumed that the issues existed between the mom and daughter. The mother brought up how the daughter was at school, but I only briefly explored that. Because relational diagnosis assumes that family relationships are the most important.

So, what is diagnosis? Diagnosis is the distillation of theory to the present micro-context. How you ask questions and gather information reflects your theory, its hypotheses, and the assumptions on which it's built. The description you provide or category you choose based on the information you gather is the application of theory to the phenomena of interest. Diagnosis, in family therapy, is the activity of gathering information to describe and explain what is going on with the clients in front of you.

The purpose of a diagnosis in family therapy is to set the stage for effective intervention. If we can adequately describe what is going on in our clients' lives, then we can know how and when to intervene. If we have a bad diagnosis, then it's likely that our intervention will be ineffective.

The validity of your diagnosis in family therapy relies on two factors – the validity of your theory and your knowledge of that theory. If diagnosis is the application of theory, then if the theory is bad the diagnosis is bad. Throughout history there have been some pretty bad theories, leading to some bad diagnoses, and bad interventions. Hippocrates' theory of the human body proposed that there were four substances – blood, phlegm, black bile, and yellow bile. Using this theory, doctors of his era would diagnosis disease by figuring out in which substance the problem existed. In many cases, it was decided that the problem was in the blood. From that, the intervention of bloodletting was created. If the problem was in the blood, letting out the bad blood would cure the patient. Needless to say, this intervention was ineffective.

Another bad theory is the theory of heteronormativity. Historically and currently, many people believe that healthy relationships can only occur in straight relationships. If you are in any other type of relationship, the theory suggests, you can't be happy. This theory led many doctors and therapists to diagnose gay and lesbian relationships as pathological. Because of this diagnosis, they created conversion therapy as a way to "cure" someone of their "gay disease." This intervention, based on bad theory and poor diagnosis, has caused tremendous amounts of unnecessary suffering.

Good theory can also lead to bad diagnosis. If the person making the diagnosis isn't well-versed in theory, it's likely that their diagnosis will reflect that. The diagnosis will be incomplete or inadequate because it's based on an incomplete or inadequate understanding of the theory. Herein lies one of the crucial problems of fusing theory, diagnosis, and intervention together. If you don't teach them as distinct elements of family therapy, then we can never develop the expertise necessary to diagnose well. If the purpose of diagnosis in family therapy is to set the stage for intervention, then poor diagnosis is going to result in bad intervention.

Intervention in Family Therapy

What Is Intervention? And What Is the Purpose of Intervention in Family Therapy?

Intervention is what we do in therapy to shape, challenge, or change the lives of clients in therapy. If there is a problem, we intervene to try and alleviate it. If there is conflict, we try to work through it. Intervention can sometimes look a lot like diagnosis. Therapists may often ask questions while intervening. But the questions asked to diagnose are different than the ones asked to intervene. Diagnostic questions are about gaining information about the clients. Intervention questions are about trying to shift the conversation or interaction to deal with the issue presented.

The purpose of intervention in family therapy is to create change and generate growth. Specifically, the purpose of intervention is built on assumptions of family therapy theories. If family therapy theories assume that the family is the context of human suffering and flourishing, the purpose of intervention is to help people cope with and grow through suffering so they can flourish. If family therapy theories assume that the quality of our relationships determines the quality of our lives, the purpose of intervention is to foster loving relationships.

Collections of interventions in family therapy are called models. Sometimes interventions in one model are found in interventions in another model. But specific collections of interventions are often given different names because the decision to include or exclude specific interventions is based upon the theory on which the model is built. For example, Structural Family Therapy is an intervention model based on family systems theory. The collection of interventions found in Structural Family Therapy is all about shifting processes and power in the family. Emotionally focused therapy for couples (EFT) is an intervention model based on attachment theory. The collection of interventions in this model aims to create emotional safety and trust.

Models aren't theory, but the theory on which the model is built provides the framework to decide which interventions are important and which aren't. Models aren't diagnosis, but often the theory that underlies the model is the same one that underlies the diagnosis. The possible diagnoses that exist in each theory are connected to the collections of interventions in the model. You wouldn't intervene in something that you can't diagnosis. In other words, if your theory suggests that the diagnosis of depression is not valid, then you wouldn't develop interventions to alleviate the symptoms of depression.

Rethinking the Trinity

In the preceding sections, I've defined theory, diagnosis, and intervention and talked about the purpose of each in family therapy. But I want to make the contrasts and connections between the three even clearer. I want to discuss how theory, diagnosis, and intervention are typically understood in family therapy, and why this creates problems in reaching, teaching, and doing therapy. Then I'll argue how I see them. I'm going to spend time detailing why I think the differences between these two representations of the family therapy trinity are important, and I'll argue why I think my take helps us train better family therapists and do better therapy.

Second, I want to walk you through a hypothetical supervision meeting between me and a student. I want to show you how conceptualizing theory, diagnosis, and intervention as separate entities with different but connected purposes can help us do better therapy. My hope is that through this exercise the arguments I'm making can be better exemplified.

The Problem With Consubstantiation

In order to rethink the trinity of family therapy, I want to return to our earlier discussion of the holy trinity. If you'll look at Figure 3.1, you'll see a depiction of the consubstantiation of the trinity in theology. Theologians and philosophers often use this representation to explain the trinity (or at least Wikipedia does).

This illustration suggests the following statements about the trinity:

1. The Father is God.
2. The Son is God.
3. The Holy Spirit is God.
4. The Father is not the Son.
5. The Father is not the Holy Spirit.
6. The Son is not the Holy Spirit.

But if you look carefully, you'll see that some of these statements are contradictory. Do you remember learning about the transitive property in one of your math classes? The transitive property is simple. It means that A = B and B = C then A = C. Or to spell it out, if two things are equal to another thing, then those two things must also be equal. In this case if the Father = God, and the Son = God, then that means that the Father = Son. In other words, because of the transitive property, these statements must also be true:

1. The Father is the Son.
2. The Father is the Holy Spirit.
3. The Son is the Holy Spirit.

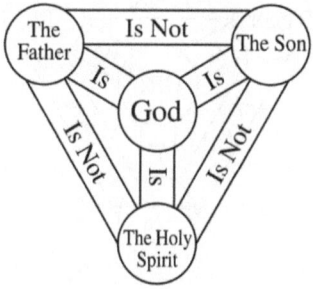

Figure 3.1 Theological representation of consubstantiation

I'm not going to debate the theological accuracy of these statements. If you want to read more about them, I suggest looking at Dale Tuggy's work (e.g., Tuggy, 2013). He dives into that debate well.

But I think this illustrates visually how we typically understand theory, diagnosis, and intervention in family therapy. If you'll look at Figure 3.2, I doctored the theological figure and replaced them with the terms we are interested in here. This model has the same logical problems as the original figure.

Specifically, it means that all the following statements are true.

1. Theory is family therapy.
1. Diagnosis is family therapy.
2. Intervention is family therapy.
3. Theory is not diagnosis.
4. Theory is not intervention.
5. Diagnosis is not intervention.
6. Theory is diagnosis.
7. Theory is intervention.
8. Diagnosis is intervention.

To me these statements illustrate the current understanding of theory, diagnosis, and intervention in family therapy. They are all the same thing but not the same thing, yet also the same thing.

Those who support the consubstantial view of theory, diagnosis, and intervention argue that they are typically doing all these things at once. In other words, they are the same and not the same because I can be asking a question that is both about diagnosis and an intervention. Or when I'm using my theory to filter the information the client is giving me to create a diagnosis, I'm also interviewing because I can use the theory to challenge my clients to shift their interactions through my questions.

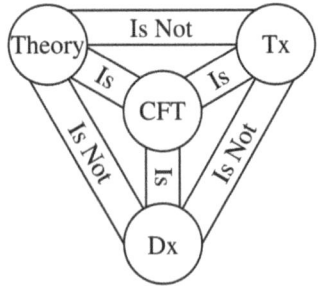

Figure 3.2 Representation of consubstantiation in couple and family therapy. Tx = intervention; CFT = couple and family therapy; DX = diagnosis

Maybe there are some people who do this effectively. But if you extrapolate the research around multitasking to family therapy, we might be falling short. Evidence suggests that when we try to do multiple things that require attention at the same time, we don't do them well (e.g., Ngo et al., 2022). I would argue that theory, diagnosis, and intervention all require a therapist's attention. If we are doing, or assuming we are doing them all at the same time, it might be that we aren't doing them as well as we think.

What's more, if we can do theory, diagnosis, and intervention at the same time, and if they are different but the same, then how do we study them? For decades models of family therapy have been developed. The creators of these models seem to always argue that their new model is better than old models. But when we put two models head-to-head, we typically see no difference between the outcomes of either model (citation). This has led to endless debates about common factors of therapy and models of intervention (citation) – arguments that have done little to move the field forward.

But other disciplines, not related to psychotherapy, do things differently. Because they see theory, diagnosis, and intervention as distinct they see leaps in their theories. This results in a better explanation of the thing in front of them, and better technologies to make life better. Let's use physics as an example. Physicists have long theorized about space, time, and motion. And this has resulted in better explanations of the world around us, which in turn has led to advancements in technologies that in many cases make our lives better.

One of the most well-known theories of physics was developed in the 17th century by Isaac Newton. Newton's theory of physics is as known as the "three laws of motion" and the "law of gravitation." This theory had hypotheses about matter, energy, and the interaction between them. Newton, and other researchers, used this theory to explain and predict many things. These laws accurately explained the movement of the stars and planets, but also created technology that we often don't associate with physics. For example, some have argued that Newton's work gave rise to the industrial revolution (Bekar & Lipsey, 2004). They have argued that Newton's ideas of motion gave rise not only to knowledge but to the cultural desire to mechanize production processes.

Newton's ideas brought about great progress – not only in motion but in explaining light, electricity, and magnetism. But many of his ideas were debunked by new data that came about in the 19th century. In fact, the work of physicists in the 19th century created so many advancements that Albert Michelson, the first U.S. citizen to win a Nobel Prize in science, argued that there was little more to learn and that the current theory and understanding of physics could be used to explain "all the phenomena which comes under our notice" (University of Chicago,

1896). But just like those who thought Newton's theory explained it all, the 20th century would again see new and better theories.

What happened in the early 20th century? Albert Einstein happened. Einstein's theory of relativity upended most of the work of the 19th century. Einstein's theory describes gravity as resulting when a mass distorts spacetime, rather than force acting over distance as Newton had proposed. Einstein's theory was confirmed through many experiments (e.g., Touboul et al., 2022). With new theory, came new ways to explain phenomena which led to new technologies. If you've ever used Google Maps, you have Albert Einstein to thank – at least in part.

The continued growth of physics relies on seeing theory, research, and innovation as separate but connected processes. In physics, you have theoretical physicists, applied physicists, and those who take the knowledge gained through theory and application to create new technologies. Without each or any of these, it may be that we would still be using Newton's theory to explain gravity and motion – and have very inaccurate Google Maps.

Since most family therapists lump theory, diagnosis, and intervention together, our theories haven't progressed, nor has our ability to diagnose or intervene. As such, over the last decades we haven't seen huge increases in our ability to alleviate mental health or relationship issues (e.g., Wittenborn & Holtrop, 2022). And I'm not aware of any evidence that suggests that family therapists of today do family therapy any better than family therapists from 50 years ago. The consubstantial view of theory, diagnosis, and intervention has gotten us stuck in the Newtonian stage of family therapy. To move forward, we need a different view of theory, diagnosis, and intervention in family therapy. A different view of the family therapy trinity would allow us to advance the science and application of our work.

Three Separate Entities – One Purpose

So, let's go with the Mormons on this one. As I mentioned in the beginning of this chapter, the argument made why Mormons aren't Christian stems from their view of the trinity. In Mormon theology, the Father, Son, and Holy Spirit aren't the same substance – they aren't consubstantial. Rather, Mormons believe that God, Jesus, and the Holy Spirit are separate entities; they each have distinct roles, but the roles are connected for the same purpose. Again, I'm not saying that I agree with this theological argument but to move family therapy forward, we need to reform our view of the trinity. We need to see the family therapy trinity like Mormons see the holy trinity – as three separate entities.

The family therapy trinity – theory, diagnosis, and intervention – isn't consubstantial; these three things are distinct. While each contributes to family therapy, they each have different roles. When we blur them together, the role that each plays in effective practice gets lost. To make this argument clearer, I want to distill the comments I made earlier about theory, diagnosis, and intervention into definitive statements about the trinity of family therapy. I'm going to list them out, and then I'll spend some time detailing my rationale for each:

1. Theory is the foundation of family therapy.
2. Theory circumscribes the explanations that are possible.
3. Theory sets the parameters for diagnosis and intervention.
4. Diagnosis is the application of theory to the immediate context.
5. Diagnosis explains and predicts the past, present, and future.
6. Diagnosis is the bridge between theory and intervention.
7. Intervention is the assumed remedy for the diagnosis.
8. Intervention is how we alter the present and future.

Theory is the foundation of family therapy. You can't have a branch of science, a clinical practice, or any knowledge system without theory. Knowledge, clinical practice, and science all require explanations, and explanations are not possible without theory. Every time you explain something, you are explaining it based on your theory – whether you realize it or not. If we can't explain a phenomenon, we can't comprehend it. Theory allows us to comprehend and thereby explain what is going on.

Theory circumscribes the explanations that are possible. Theory is purposefully limiting. Theory sets boundaries around the explanations that are possible and the explanations that aren't. If you've ever heard a person explain something and you thought, "that's impossible," it's probably because the boundaries of your theory are very different from the other person's. If any explanation is possible, you don't have a theory, or a way to coherently comprehend something. Without theory to say what is possible and what is not, there is no way to develop explanations or predictions.

Theory sets the parameters for diagnosis and intervention. Because theory is limiting, what stems from theory is also limiting. If theory limits possible explanations, then diagnosis and interventions that are derived from that theory are also limited. You can't diagnose something that is outside the parameters of your theory. If a certain explanation is impossible within your theory, then it can't be used to make sense of what is going on in the immediate context. And you can't intervene in something that doesn't exist. In other words, if parent-child relational problems aren't a rationale diagnosis because of the parameters of your theory, intervening to improve the parent-child relationships wouldn't make sense. In family therapy, theory tells us what the problem is and what is not.

Diagnosis is the application of theory to the immediate context. Although theory is limiting, if it's a good theory it can describe multiple patterns of the phenomena it is meant to explain. Good family therapy theory would be able to explain and predict patterns across any family. Bad family therapy theory would only be able to explain patterns in certain families. Diagnosis is applying family therapy theory to a specific family. Using a theory, therapists develop predictions and explanations of the families that come into their offices. Theory sets the parameters for diagnosis and allows therapists to use those parameters to comprehend what is going on in the families.

Diagnosis explains and predicts the past, present, and future. If you were to go to the doctor and receive a diagnosis of hypertension, this diagnosis may tell you what your current problem is, but it also provides explanations of the past and predicts what will happen in the future. If you get a diagnosis of hypertension, it can help explain why in the past you may have had unexplainable headaches in the morning, or nosebleeds, or even chest pains or muscle tremors. What's more the doctor is also predicting that you likely smoked or consumed too much alcohol, or that your ancestors passed down genes that put you at greater risk, or that you aren't exercising or eating well. The doctor is also saying that without intervention, the future could hold greater problems – heart attack or stroke. Diagnosis in family therapy does the same. When we apply theory to a specific family, we are making predictions and explanations about what has transpired in the past, what is happening now, and what will happen in the future.

Diagnosis is the bridge between theory and intervention. I mentioned this earlier but to reiterate it: you can't treat what you can't diagnosis, and you can't diagnose what you can't explain. When family therapists say that they don't "believe in diagnosis," what they are saying is that they don't need an explanation to intervene. It's the assumption that the intervention itself is sufficient. While that may work in some instances, it can become problematic in others. In many instances if you intervene without a theory or diagnosis, you make ad hoc explanations. Often ad hoc explanations end up dismissing important or contradictory information. If you intervene without theory or diagnosis, you may end up helping your clients but trying to replicate that with other clients most likely won't work. That is why diagnosis is so important. It provides the connection between your theory and your intervention. It allows you to say, "I did this because . . ." Without a diagnosis to tie theory and intervention together, explanations of "because" are made up after the fact.

Intervention is the assumed remedy for the diagnosis. The reason family therapists intervene is because they assume that the intervention will be helpful. But what is helpful and what is not, is determined by theory. In other words, your intervention can only remedy what is possible to diagnose within your theory. And the theory dictates what is a good outcome. For example, in couples therapy, much of the time an intervention is deemed successful only if the partners stay together. Part of every diagnosis, then, is that patterns that lead to the possible disintegration of a couple relationship are problematic. Your intervention is going to work toward the goal of changing the patterns that pull the couple apart and amplify those patterns that pull them together. Your success is often determined if you have remedied the threat of separation. However, if the theory and diagnosis are different, the remedy and outcomes must also change. If you are working with a couple and diagnose one partner with depression this changes what outcome is considered successful. Your intervention may separate the couple, but if the depression symptoms are improved, then therapy could be deemed successful.

Intervention is how we alter the present and future. Diagnosis explains the past and present and predicts the future. Intervention allows us to change it. If you go back to the earlier example of hypertension, if the person with hypertension is given medication to lower their blood pressure; if they begin exercising and change their diet; and if they quit smoking or lessen their alcohol intake, their risk of stroke or heart attack decreases. The same is true for intervention in family therapy. If we can diagnosis effectively, we can create interventions or collections of interventions that can alter the course of the diagnosis.

These statements don't reflect everything that can or will be written about the family therapy trinity but are the main points of the argument I am trying to make. Yes, theory, diagnosis, and intervention are connected. But they are not the same. Each has a distinct role and purpose in family therapy. Theory is the foundation and driver of family therapy. Diagnosis is how we understand what is going on with our clients. Intervention is how we alter what will happen. We have to combine these powers to produce the best possible outcomes.

Let's see how this might play out in a supervision setting. I'm going to make up a dialogue between me and a supervisee I'll call Joyce. Let's assume Joyce is a 2nd year PhD student who is working with a couple in our program's clinic. The couple – Gary and Adam – have been married since 2004. They have two kids, ages 18 and 16. Gary and Adam came to Joyce because they felt distance in their relationship, and they wanted it fixed before their kids left for college. They are worried that if they don't address the growing distance between them, there may not be much left when their kids move out. Joyce has seen Gary and Adam for six sessions, but she is bringing them up in supervision because she feels stuck.

Supervisor: Ok, so tell me a bit more about what you've been working on with Gary and Adam.

Joyce: Well, they wanted greater connection, so we've been working on trying to get them to share their emotions in ways that bring them closer together.

Supervisor: And how is that going?

Joyce: It was going well at first, but then it felt like everything blew up. They ended up getting into a huge fight after one of our sessions, so now we have just been rehashing the same fight over and over again.

Supervisor: So, therapy over the past few weeks has just been about the fight?

Joyce: Yeah, I feel like something about this fight was hurtful or important, but I just can't seem to make sense of it. They said that this fight felt different, but when I try to ask them why, they can't really explain it. I've tried to slow them down a bit, but they end up getting frustrated in session because they think I'm not getting it and that maybe therapy is making it worse.

Supervisor: What theory have you been grounding your work in?

Joyce: Well, I've been using EFT, so we've been doing lots of emotional expanding and enactments to try and help them shift their cycle.

Supervisor: Hold on just a second. When I say theory, I'm not wanting to know how you are intervening, I'm wanting to know what theory you are using to conceptualize Gary and Adam's relationship.

Joyce: Ok, yeah, I mean EFT is based on attachment theory, so I guess the theory I'm using would be attachment theory.

Supervisor: Great. And what is attachment theory as you understand it? What are the core assumptions or hypotheses of attachment theory?

Joyce: Attachment theory is about bonding. It assumes that humans need each other to have happy and successful lives. It's about building trust and security.

Supervisor: Yes, and why do humans need trust and security in their relationships?

Joyce: I mean, they need a secure base from which to explore the world. If they don't have a safe place to go when they are stressed, they won't venture out. If they don't think that anyone is going to be there when they reach for them, it becomes isolating.

Supervisor: Exactly. A secure base is a key tenet of attachment theory. What else?

Joyce: Well, the flip side of a secure base is an insecure base. If we are connected to someone that is unpredictable, or untrustworthy, we end up feeling insecure in the world around us.

Supervisor: Yes. Security and insecurity are key ideas of attachment theory. And how do we learn if a connection is secure or insecure?

Joyce: Through interactions. If we reach for someone and they respond to us in a way that makes us feel safe – and this happens over and over again – we have created a secure bond with that person. If we reach for someone and they aren't there when we need them, we can get anxious or shut down. If this happens over and over again, we may start believing that there is something wrong with us – that we aren't worthy of connection, or that there is something wrong with the other person.

Supervisor: How would this understanding of attachment theory help you to explain what is going on with Gary and Adam? How could we use attachment theory to diagnose what has happened in their relationships?

Joyce: Hmmm, well, I think that something that was once secure has become insecure.

Supervisor: Say more about that.

Joyce: When they describe the early parts of their relationship – before they got married and before they had kids – they talk about it really fondly. In some ways they get frustrated because it seems that they have lost what they had before.

Supervisor: Right, so what have they lost? What was there once that no longer is?

Joyce: Well, in the simplest terms the secure base. They used to be each other's secure base, but that has gone away.

Supervisor: Ok. What was happening between Gary and Adam when their relationship was secure?

Joyce: I haven't really talked about that with them. We've just really been focused on the crisis at hand.

Supervisor: Ok, well, if they lost their secure base, what has replaced it?

Joyce: I guess an insecure relationship.

Supervisor: And what makes this relationship insecure? What happens within and between the couple that creates insecurity?

Joyce: Well, they very much have a pursuer-distancer relationship. That's what really drives their insecurity.

Supervisor: Break down this pursuer-distancer pattern. And when you do, let's not forget the theory that can help us diagnosis this issue.

Joyce: Attachment theory, right. Adam is really the one that reaches out. He tends to try and make a connection with Gary – to feel more connected, safer – but often he does this in a way that Gary reacts poorly to. Gary will feel like Adam is too needy or just complaining about things that aren't necessary. Gray tries to shut down the conversation and if he can't, he tends to just shut himself down.

Supervisor: So is this the same pattern that got them into the big fight you talked about?

Joyce: Yeah, except that instead of Gary just shutting down, he ended up getting really angry and yelling.

Supervisor: And has this ever happened before? This variation of their insecure pattern?

Joyce: I'm not sure. We haven't really talked about Gary getting angry, we've really just talked about the main pattern.

Supervisor: Well, what do you think you still need to know to better diagnose what's going on with this latest change in their relationship?

Joyce: I think I might need to first get more information about their history as a couple and as people.

Supervisor: And why would this be important from an attachment theory perspective?

Joyce: Well, attachment theory suggests that we tend to replicate patterns in a previous attachment relationship. So, if I can better understand some of their previous attachment relationships, it might help contextualize what is going on currently.

Supervisor: Great, and what else?

Joyce: I think I want to know about the evolution of their attachment relationship. If it was good in the beginning, how did it change? Attachment theory would argue that secure relationships can change as the people in them change, so that might be important.

Supervisor: Exactly. If you are using attachment theory to frame your diagnosis, this is all going to be valuable information. Is there anything else you think attachment theory might want you to explore?

Joyce: Hmmm, well, I don't know much about their relationships with their kids, but I would assume that those are important attachment relationships to them. It could be that these relationships are helping to shape the move from a secure relationship to an insecure one.

Supervisor: I think that's a good idea. Another idea might be exploring how unsafe their world is. By that I mean, the secure base hypothesis suggests that if we feel safe with someone we can better navigate a world that is unpredictable. Right now, there is lots of threats to Gary and Adam's marriage – some people are very hostile to gay marriage.

Joyce: Yeah, I mean they have talked about that stress – especially given the political climate in Iowa right now. But we haven't really spent time fleshing that out.

Supervisor: It sounds to me that there is a bit more to explore to really get a grasp of what is going on for them.

Joyce: Agreed. I think that this gives me a bunch of ideas and topics to explore with them. I think once I get a better handle on what has happened, it'll be easier to see what is getting us stuck.

Supervisor: I think so too. And it may help you better understand why they weren't responding to the interventions that you were trying with them. It also might be good to revisit some of the things you read about attachment theory. It might help you find additional avenues to explore that really might help with the diagnosis.

Joyce: I was thinking the same thing.

This example is overly simple. Often discussions that take place in supervision aren't as neat and tidy as this. But I hope this example allows you to clearly understand the arguments I've been making in this chapter. Theory, diagnosis, and intervention are important components of family therapy – but they are not the same. They need and rely on each other, but they all have different purposes. However, the drive of both diagnosis and intervention is theory. The validity of our diagnosis and the effectiveness of our interventions are only as good as our theory. There are competing theories in family therapy – in the supervision example the theory being used was attachment theory. But I'm going to argue for a specific theory: family systems theory.

The next chapter is all about family systems. What it is and what it isn't. I'm going to outline the epistemology and assumptions on which it is built and talk about the tenets and hypotheses. I'm going to argue that family systems theory, based on the currently available evidence, is the best theory on which to diagnose. I'm not going to have the space to lay out all the evidence for family systems theory – and I've done that in my previous book, *The Science of Family Systems Theory*. So, to really get an in-depth view of the evidence, I suggest spending some time evaluating the evidence I present in that book. But before we jump into family systems theory, I want to be clear about my arguments regarding theory, diagnosis, and intervention. Next, I've summarized what I see as the core arguments of this chapter.

Recap: Main Ideas and Arguments

1. **In family therapy, we often conflate theory, diagnosis, and intervention.** This has narrowed our ability to practice. When we conflate theory, diagnosis, and intervention, we end up doing none of them well. To advance the field and to build better diagnosis and intervention models we need to be clear about the purpose and role of theory, diagnosis, and intervention.
2. **Theory is the foundation of family therapy.** We use theory in family therapy to circumscribe explanations, and set the parameters for diagnosis and intervention.
3. **Diagnosis is the application of theory to the immediate context.** We use theory to make diagnostic statements about the past,

present, and future. Diagnosis bridges theory and intervention. Without diagnosis, you can't link theory to intervention.

4. **Intervention is the assumed remedy for the diagnosis – it allows therapists to alter the present and the future.** The goal of family therapy has always been alleviating issues or problems that occur in families. But to effectively intervene, therapists must be able to accurately diagnose.

5. **If family therapy is going to advance, we must use and apply theory, diagnosis, and intervention as intended.** Though theory, diagnosis, and intervention are all connected, they are not the same. If therapists are going to apply them as intended, they must understand what makes them different as well as what connects them.

Chapter 4

Family Systems Theory

"What is family systems theory?" This question was the impetus for my first book, *The Science of Family Systems Theory*. As a professor at the University of Iowa, it's a question I would ask students during the oral defense of their comprehensive exams. When I'd ask it, a conversation like this one would play out:

Me: So, you wrote in your documents about clinical practice that your work is grounded in family systems theory. What is family systems theory? Or what are the main hypotheses of family systems theory?

Student: Well, family systems theory is about connections. I guess its main idea is that the whole is greater than the sum of its parts. It means that the family is more than just the people that are a part of it.

Me: Okay. Say more about that. Is the whole being greater than the sum of its parts a hypothesis? An assumption of the theory? Or something else?

Student: Well, it's more of a main idea. I guess the hypotheses are more about boundaries, and feedback loops.

Me: And what does family systems theory hypothesize about boundaries and feedback loops?

Student: Hmmm . . . I guess it's about homeostasis and isomorphism. I'm not sure I'm answering your question.

Me: Not exactly, but that's okay.

I try not to be too much of a jerk in oral defenses, so typically I'll back off at that point and start giving my spiel about theory, diagnosis, and intervention. I'll carry on and on, saying that family systems theory does have clear, testable hypotheses; that as a field we've done a poor job of teaching it; and that because of this it's stuck. If you've ever been to an oral defense, you'll notice that many professors, like me, talk way too much during them.

But I want you to ask yourself the same question – what is family systems theory? Do you have a better answer?

DOI: 10.4324/9781003295907-6

Most likely you don't.

Why? Because when we lump together theory, diagnosis, and intervention, theory can get really muddled. Roxi Chen and her colleagues (2017) looked at the use of the theory in family therapy research articles. Many articles used family systems theory but didn't define it and didn't tie the results of the study back to the theory. They would often just say that the study was "guided by family systems theory" – just like my students suggest that their clinical practice is guided by family systems theory. It's a way to talk about it without really knowing what it means.

The most comprehensive distillation of family systems theory hypotheses I've seen was done by Alan Carr in 2015. He argued for 20 family systems hypotheses. These hypotheses were classified into seven groups, each containing two or three hypotheses: 1) systems, 2) boundaries, 3) patterns, 4) stability, 5) change, 6) complexity, and 7) application. But Carr himself acknowledges the lack of clarity within these hypotheses, saying

> The propositions described above . . . derived from systems theory and cybernetics have evolved within the broad field of couple and family therapy. **They are by no means a single integrated framework. Nor are all of these propositions incorporated into all of the foundational theoretical models . . . or evidence-based clinical treatment models.** However, they do represent most of the important aspects of systems theory (bold is added).

To me, Carr is reflecting what Chen and her colleagues said – we don't really know what to talk about when we are asked to define family systems theory, so we just talk about everything. Family systems theory as typically taught and applied is an ethereal framework, not a theory.

Now, some of you may be thinking, what about Bowen's family systems theory? Didn't he lay out a clear version of family systems theory? I would argue that he did. In the book he wrote with Michael Kerr, Murray Bowen spells out a theory with testable hypotheses. But on the very first page of the book, Kerr and Bowen say something that is often forgotten by people who read it. They write:

> Family systems theory is based on the assumption that the human is a product of evolution and that human behavior is significantly regulated by the same natural processes that regulate the behavior of all other living things. . . . While developed on the assumption of the human's tie to nature, family systems theory is only a step *toward* understanding the human in this context of natural systems, since **we have barely scratched the surface on what will eventually be known about the forces that regulate the behavior of all life** (bold is added).

Kerr and Bowen wrote that in 1988. Since then, we've mapped the human genome; our understanding of the brain, nervous system, and our bodies has grown exponentially; the theory of evolution has added even more evidence to support its claims; we have a better understanding of the important processes in human family relationships; and we better understand how larger culture, power, oppression, and the systems that support them affect the family.

In 1988, we may have "barely scratched the surface" in our knowledge about what regulates human life and relationships, but I'd argue we know much more now. When we know more, our theories should be updated. In my first book, that's what I tried to do. I presented a family systems theory that had clear hypotheses and spelled out the evidence for those hypotheses. I'm not going to rehash that evidence here. But I am going to summarize the version of family systems theory I argued for in *The Science of Family Systems Theory*. To formulate systemic diagnoses, we are going to need to understand family systems theory.

But to do that, we need to answer another question first: What is a system?

What Is a System?

This is another question that I also like to ask in oral defenses. I often serve on defense committees for other disciplines. Regardless of the topic, it seems that everyone uses the word "system." They'll talk about the "school system," "the health care system," "systems of oppression," or "the nervous system." Again, I try not to be too much of a jerk, but if someone is repeatedly using the word "system," I'll ask them to define it. Typically, I'm met with stammering and blank stares.

We also use the word "system" in non-academic settings. We say things like "all systems go" or "get it out of my system." A system can be a scheme for getting what we want, or it can be something that should work but doesn't (e.g., "our political system is broken"). Regardless of how we talk about it, we typically don't really define or explain what we mean when we use the word "system."

Though "system" has been in use since the 1600s, I'm going to fast forward a couple of centuries and use the definition that Ludwig von Bertalanffy provided of "system." If you're not familiar, von Bertalanffy was a German biologist who is credited as one of the originators of general systems theory. Writing in 1968, he provided a definition of system. It's a bit complex, so read the definition and then we'll discuss it a bit more. He wrote:

> A system can be defined as a set of elements standing in interrelations. Interrelation means that elements, *p*, stand in relations, *R*, so that the behavior of an element *p* in *R* is different from its behavior

in another relation, R'. If the behaviors in R and R' are not different, there is no interaction, and the elements behave independently with respect to the relations R and R'.

Like I said, it's a bit complex so let's unpack it.

The first thing von Bertalanffy talks about is "a set of elements." Elements aren't just the ones we learn about in chemistry class. In a general systems perspective, elements can be anything that can interact with another thing. We have elements within cells that interact – like the nucleolus and cytoplasm. We have elements in our bodies that interact – like our brain and our nerves. People can be elements in a system. Groups of people that interact with other groups of people can be elements. Elephants can interact with other elephants. Planets are elements of a solar system. If a thing can interact with another thing, it's an element.

But to be a system these sets of elements must interact or interrelate in a specific way. As von Bertalanffy argues, an element that interacts with another element doesn't necessarily constitute a system. It must be different from its interaction within another relationship. In other words, the way we define the system is dependent on the way that the elements in the system interact. A system, to be a system, must have elements that have distinct interactions. The uniqueness or distinctness of these interactions is the purpose or function of the system.

To emphasize this point even more, I want to draw on a more modern take of the definition of a system. In 2008, Donella Meadows provided this definition of system. As you'll see it contains everything that von Bertalanffy described but in a bit less complex manner. Meadows wrote:

> A system isn't just an old collection of things. A system is an interconnected set of elements that is coherently organized in a way that achieves something. If you look at the definition closely for a minute, you can see that a system must consist of three kinds of things: elements, interconnections, and a function or purpose.
>
> For example, the elements of your digestive system include teeth, enzymes, stomach, and intestines. They are interrelated through the physical flow of food, and an elegant set of regulating chemical signals. The function of this system is to break down food into its basic nutrients and to transfer those nutrients into the bloodstream (another system) while discarding unusable wastes. . . .
>
> Is there anything that is not a system? Yes – a conglomeration without any particular interconnections or function. Sand scattered on a road by happenstance is not, itself, a system. You can add sand or take away sand and you still have just sand on the road. Arbitrarily add or take away football players, or pieces of your digestive system, and you quickly no longer have the same system. . . .

You can see from these examples that there is integrity or wholeness about a system and an active set of mechanisms to maintain that integrity. Systems can change, adapt, respond to events, seek goals, mend injuries, and attend to their own survival in lifelike ways, although they may consist of nonliving things. Systems can be self-organizing, and often are self-repairing over at least some range of disruptions. They are resilient, and many of them are evolutionary. Out of one system other completely new, never-before-imagined systems can arise.

Meadows provides concrete examples of von Bertalanffy's definition. Systems are comprised of interconnected elements. The patterns or rules of the interactions are unique or distinct and give the system its purpose or function.

Biological and Social Systems

While all systems have elements, interactions, and purpose, there can be important differences between types of systems. To understand family systems theory and systemic diagnosis, I want to focus on two types of systems: biological systems and social systems.

To understand biological systems, we need to look to the field of systems biology. Systems biology is founded on the idea that biological organisms are systems that have two properties – autonomy and adaptation. When systems biologists talk about autonomy they are not talking about the colloquial usage of autonomy – freedom from external control or self-governance. To the systems biologists, autonomy has a specific definition. Bernd Rosslenbroich outlined this definition in his 2014 book, *On the Origin of Autonomy*. In it, he provides this definition:

> Living systems are autonomous in the sense that they maintain themselves in form and function within time and achieve a self-determined flexibility.

He expounds on this definition by suggesting that autonomous systems:

1. *Generate, maintain, and regulate an inner network of interdependent, energy consuming processes, which in turn generate and maintain the system;*
2. *Establish a boundary and actively regulate their interactions and exchange with the environment;*
3. *Specify their own rules of behavior and react to external stimuli in a self-determined way, according to their internal disposition and condition;*

4. *Establish an interdependence between the system and its parts within the organism, which includes a differentiation in subsystems;*
5. *Establish a time autonomy; and*
6. *Maintain a phenotypic stability (robustness) in the face of diverse perturbations arising from environmental changes, internal variability, and genetic variations.*

Autonomy is about the interactions in the system – the interrelations between the elements in the system – not the elements themselves. The interactions are what create and maintain the system, and they have rules or patterns, are interdependent, and create a boundary (distinction and purpose) between the system and the environment. There is lots of jargon, in this definition, so let's simplify it a bit: Autonomy is the ability of interactions in a system to generate and maintain distinct connections between elements that give the system purpose.

Autonomy is a key property of biological systems but for a system to have autonomy it also needs the ability to adapt. Let's return to Bernd Rosslenbroich's 2014 book, *On the Origin of Autonomy*. Rosslenbroich notes that autonomy is never absolute, it's relative. A system is never wholly separate from its environment. Autonomy is dependent on the system-environment relationship. He writes:

> the internal compartment is established within a boundary, which the system generates as a spatial separation from the environment. In its simplest form, this is realized in a single-cell organism by means of a cell membrane. However, even the simple example of the cell membrane shows that in a biological system complete separation is never obtained. Instead, we see the double function of a boundary and an exchange with the environment through and across the boundary. Each cell membrane and each integument of an animal has to perform a double function.

The autonomy that serves to generate and maintain the system allows the system to distinguish itself from the environment, but at the same time this boundary is continually interacting and responding to the environment. In other words, the systems are not only autonomous, but they also are adaptable.

Rosslenbroich describes adaptation and its association with autonomy later in the book. He writes:

> Adaptedness is a relational property of an organism or rather a property of the organism-environment system. . . . [A]utonomy and adaptation become a central pair of this system. Both are dependent on each other: On the one hand, there is the organism, and on the other

hand is the environment. The organism – even in its simplest form – always establishes its life function together with the generation of a boundary and thus produces its 'being different' from the surrounding environment. To maintain this state, the organism not only needs regulatory and stabilizing functions on the one hand but needs to react appropriately to cope successfully with the environmental influences . . . autonomy needs adaptations.

If a system has autonomy, it has adapted. If the system has adapted, it has autonomy. These two properties are dependent on each other. A biological system cannot exist without autonomy and adaptation. Adaptations, then, are changes to a system's autonomy in response to the exchange the system has with its environment.

But how do systems adapt or experience changes in their autonomy? Rosslenbroich proposes a few ideas on what happens – he calls these the "set of resources to change autonomy (adapt)" or as "increasing autonomy." He doesn't see this as a complete list but sees evidence for these throughout the evolutionary history. The first resources are *spatial separation from the environment*. From a biological perspective, these include things such as cell walls, shells, hair, and skin. These features all:

> serve to keep the environment outside the organisms and to regulate and direct the exchange with it. Changes in their organization can contribute to an essential degree to changes in the organisms-environment relation.

The physical boundary a system generates to keep them separate from their environment helps keep the system and the environment separate. But to maintain that separateness, the boundary must regulate exchanges with the environment. When the environment changes, the system must adapt.

The second resource is the *homeostatic functions* of the system. While there can be multiple, Rosslenbroich talks about two: homeostasis and robustness. Rosslenbroich defines homeostasis as "the ability of a system to regulate its internal conditions to keep some or several functions stable," and robustness as "the property that allows a system to maintain its functions against internal and external perturbations and uncertainties." These homeostatic functions allow a system to be resistant to the environment. If a system adapts too quickly to changes, it may lose its autonomy.

Internalization is another resource to change autonomy. Internalization happens when a function that typically occurred outside the system gets brought inside the system. Rosslenbroich argues that this type of adaptation has been seen throughout evolutionary history. One example is the evolution from gills to lungs. Gills were a part of the way that an organism regulated the exchange with the environment, allowing air inside the body. As changes in the environments and in organisms occurred, this process was internalized – it was literally moved from the outside (gills) to the inside (lungs) of organisms.

A *gain in size* is the second resource for changing autonomy. When a function is internalized, there needs to be more physical space to allow for that function – lungs tend to take up more room than gills. But gaining size can also give the system many benefits including greater control over homeostatic functions. What's more, if you are bigger, then you are less likely to be eaten by things that are smaller than you.

Finally, Rosslenbroich suggests that *flexibility within the environment* is another resource changing autonomy. He writes:

> prerequisites for establishing a certain amount of physiological flexibility within a given environment, that is, a capability of organism to generate flexible functional answers to conditions and changes in their environment . . . these principles can be widened to include all forms of behavioral flexibility, emancipating organisms from mere short-term reactions to environmental factors. Together, these elements are able to generate certain degrees of physiological and behavioral freedom.

In other words, if a system has something that separates it from the environment, it has room to internalize functions, it's going to have better control of its homeostasis and robustness, giving it more freedom over its physiological and behavioral reactions to the environment.

Rosslenbroich categorizes these ideas into two dimensions: interactive autonomy and constructive autonomy. He writes:

> Increasing autonomy is defined as an evolutionary shift in the system-environment relationship, such that direct influences of the environment on the respective individual systems are gradually reduced (interactive autonomy) and stability and flexibility of self-referential, intrinsic functions within the systems are generated and enhanced (constitutive autonomy).

Interactive autonomy are those factors that reduce the effect, influence, or power that the environment has on the system. Constitutive autonomy is the enhancement of the intrinsic systemic interactions or processes that provide stability and flexibility for the system.

In writing about evolution and adaptation, others have echoed these two main ideas of interactive and constitutive dimensions of increasing autonomy. However, they include an additional dimension as well.

Specifically, writing in their book, *Biological Autonomy*, Alvaro Moreno and Matteo Mossio (2015) argue for a third dimension, the historical dimension. They write:

> Autonomy . . . lies at the intersection between different dimensions, and specifically the constitutive and interactive ones. . . . Yet this isn't the whole story; autonomy also has a *historical* dimension . . . no adequate understanding of the emergence of an autonomous system can be obtained without taking into account the evolutionary processes that brought them about.

In other words, the interactive and constitutive dimensions of adaptation tell us about the current adaptive or adapting state of a system which gives the system its autonomy, while the historical dimension traces how the system has adapted in the past. For a system to maintain autonomy, it must increase or respond to the environment over time. In other words, to exist in the present, the system has adapted in the past.

Again, there is a lot of jargon that I've thrown at you, so let's take a beat and summarize the main ideas that you'll need to make a systemic diagnosis. Autonomy and adaptation are symbiotic – in biological systems you can't have one without the other. Biological systems are autonomous systems – they have interactions that serve to generate and maintain the system. In other words, elements in a system must interact or there is no system. For a system to continue over time it must adapt. Adaptation is a shift in the system-environment relationship. This happens in two dimensions – the interactive dimension and the constitutive dimension. The system-environment relationships change by changing how the system interacts with the environment (the interactive dimension) and this is done be changing the autonomy generating interactions making them more flexible or more stable (the constitutive dimension).

We can't understand the present adaptive and adapting state of an autonomous system without understanding how it has developed. The historical dimension of a system traces how a system has changed its relationship with the environment by making changes in the interactive and constitutive dimensions. Biological systems have autonomy and change or increase their autonomy by adapting. To adapt, there need to be resources that allow changes in autonomy. These resources can evolve as a system continues to interact and regulate exchanges with its environment.

With an understanding of biological systems, let's turn to social systems. To get a definition of social system, let's turn to another disciple: sociology. The idea of social systems in the field of sociology stems from Niklas Luhmann. He first published his book, *Social Systems*, in 1984.

Since that time others have built on his work, but many of his ideas remain valid and are key definitions of social systems.

Luhmann argued that, like biological systems, social systems were autonomous – they had distinct yet adaptable processes that served to generate and maintain themselves. But unlike biological systems, social systems are created by operations that exist as passing events. Writing about Luhmann's work in 2018, Jean-Sébastien Guy, described this as follows:

> [Luhmann] abandoned the classical definition of a systems as a 'whole made out of parts.' For him, a system involves multiple operations at the same time, yet these operations are not like Lego blocks that could be taken apart and reassembled to create a different shape. Lego blocks have lasting existence; operations do not. . . . Thus, a system is like a self-sustaining chain or cascade of events. What is important is not for the system to be copied (reproduced) as it is from one moment to the next, as if the system had to be protected against change. What matters is to maintain the capacity to continue generating more events, so that the system as a chain of operations never comes to a dead-end.

Like biologicals systems, social systems sustain themselves through interactions; but, unlike biological systems, the social system doesn't necessarily have the same elements all the time in each system. Rather, social systems need new interactions and new elements to be perpetual so that they remain relevant and ongoing.

Guy (2018) further expands on this idea:

> It is not necessary for the same social actors to continue pursuing the same objectives for the same social process to continue unfolding across time. For the same social processes to extend indefinitely, a chain can be created between actors so that one actor can leave the scene to be replaced with another actor without delay. Soldiers die on the battlefield, but the war still goes on as new recruits are sent to the front. In Luhmann's theory, the same applies for art, law, science, religion, etc. Each of these systems (or subsystems) is like a process that has been going on for many centuries already, a process that does not progress toward an ultimate end . . . but that perpetually transforms itself to survive both the passage of time and the passing of social actors. . . . Social systems are always-in-the-making, continuously remaking themselves.

One clear example of this can be seen in the social system of racial hierarchy and racism in the United States. From chattel slavery starting in 1619, to Jim Crow law enacted after the Civil War, to housing and education segregation law in the early part of the 20th century, to drug policies that led to mass incarceration in the late 20th and early 21st centuries, to present day measures to restrict voting rights, the system of racism has transformed to survive the passing of time and the passing of different social actors.

But what are social systems trying to maintain? They aren't trying to pass along genes per se, nor ensuring the survival of offspring. Rather, socials systems are concerned with power and authority, and the resources that flow from that power.

Another sociologist, Max Weber, provided clear definitions and examples of power and authority. He defined power as the ability to exercise one's will over others and authority as accepted power, or power that people follow or organize around (Weber, 2002). When a person or system has access to power, and other persons or systems legitimize that power, then those in power can use their authority to allot resources. Resources that systems in power have can be material (e.g., food, water, shelter, or access to health care), but they can also be abstract (e.g., deference, acceptance, or respect).

But how do social systems maintain their access to power? Luhmann argued that it is through communication and conflict. In their book, *Unlocking Luhmann* (2021), Claudio Baraldi, Giancarlo Corsi, and Elana Eposito use the work of Luhmann to provide definitions of each of these concepts. Each of these concepts is necessary for a social system to maintain its power and authority. Let's start by talking about communication.

According to Luhmann, communication is:

> the basic element and operation of the social system. It consists of the unity of the difference among three selections: utterance, information, and understanding the difference between utterance and information.
>
> Communication is achieved if information (e.g., today it is raining) and the participant's responsibility for uttering it (saying that today it is raining) are understood as different selections. Without such understandings, there is no communication. . . . Therefore, in communication information is produced, rather than transmitted: information is not lost by someone and gained by someone else, but is uttered by someone and understood by someone else. . . .
>
> . . . an utterance of information is a selection. Utterance of information shows intentions, motives, reasons, and knowledge. It shows responsibility for speaking and for the reasons for speaking (e.g., by saying that it is raining, the speaker is answering a question, or trying to make it clear that she would like to stay home). However, utterance

of information isn't communication in itself, as understanding is the selection that realizes communication. Understanding draws a distinction between information (today it is raining) and utterance (the reason why the interlocutor says that today it is raining). The realization of communication requires the understanding of this difference, between information and (responsibility for) its utterance.

. . . social systems use communication as a specific operation for autopoietic reproduction, and the continuation of communication achieves the autopoiesis of a social system. Social systems have communication as their basic operation and include only communication. An important consequence is that individuals are not included in social systems; rather, they are systems in the environment of social systems.

I want to highlight three important points Luhmann is making. First, in social systems, communications are the elements. Communication is produced by other elements in other systems, but in a social system, communications are elements. Second, communications are also the purpose or function of social systems. In other words, because social systems are self-sustaining, their purpose is just to continue the creation of the elements – to continue the communication that replicates access to power. Finally, in a social system people are not the elements, but the social system is the environment in which people exist.

Conflict is another element of social systems. Luhmann described conflict as:

a parasite social system that requires the communication of a contradiction, and tends to absorb the resources of the system in which it develops. This is where the danger lies for the host system. The system, which hosts to the parasitic conflict, is thus faced with the necessity to keep it within acceptable boundaries.

. . . The ability of society to facilitate and tolerate conflict is by all accounts an essential requirement of its evolution. On the other hand, conflicts rapidly grow to escape the control of the host social system, creating problems and interrupting communication, the consequences of which may not be positive. In older societies based on interaction, it was therefore necessary to suppress conflict. To do so, certain roles were differentiated for the purpose – for instance, notable citizens were given the responsibility of resolving disagreements. The stratification of society permitted instead the strengthening of particular differences drawn from the conflict.

Contradictions fulfill a warning and alarm function in that they signal an inappropriateness of the system structures. They are regarded as an immune system that functions to protect the autopoietic reproduction of social systems. They warn the system that it could disappear due to internal disturbances triggered by the environment, whilst the conflict-generating *no* allows the system's reaction even without complete knowledge of the environment and the factors endangering the system itself.

This is a little complex, so let's again highlight three important points. First, conflict is the communication of contradiction. A social system runs into conflict when communication that contradicts the social system's message is produced. For example, the exclusion of gay and lesbian couples from marriage in the United States was maintained by a social system where the communication being produced was "marriage is between a husband and a wife." However, this message was contradicted by the message "love is love."

Second, when a contradiction of communication occurs, the social system must respond, or its existence is threatened. This can be done by suppressing the conflict. The system creates new communications that advocate for certain people to be in power – creating stratifications and hierarchical structures. Those to whom social system communication gives power, they adapt their message to try and maintain power. In the case of marriage, the communication becomes "marriage between a man and a woman is ordained by God." This message is the same as before, but it is using the structures it has created to try and suppress the contradictory communication that "love is love."

Finally, not all social systems suppress conflict. When used correctly, as Luhmann argues, contradictions can act as an immune system that can help the social system change the structures it supports. If the system can successfully adapt, the system evolves. Problems can arise if the system evolves too quickly, but if the system just says "no" and refuses to adapt this is also problematic.

Biological and social systems have important properties and features. Though they have different elements, interactions, and purposes, they are both systems. The properties of these two types of systems are going to be important to apply family systems theory through systemic diagnosis. But before we jump into the theory itself, we need to understand how the descriptions of biological and social systems used here frame the assumptions on which family systems theory is built.

The Assumptions of Family Systems Theory

If you remember, in the previous chapter, we discussed how all theories are built on assumptions. All theories of family therapy are built on the assumption that family relationships are key to our health and well-being. But family systems theory is built on an additional assumption that separates it from other family therapy theories: *Family systems theory assumes that the family is a biological system.*

Now some of you reading this might disagree. You might be thinking, "the family communicates and has conflicts and contradictions, so it's a social system." There are good arguments out there that could support that claim. But let's look again at what Luhmann wrote:

> in a social system people are not the elements, but the social system is the environment in which people exist.

His argument is that people are not the elements of the social system. People are biological systems – they are autonomous and adaptable. Social systems are the environment in which people exist. They are one of the systems that create the environments that human systems respond to. Human systems, including the family, create and perpetuate these social systems, but they are not elements of this system. And I agree with him.

If the family is a social system and not a biological system, then the biological systems that create the family system don't matter. In other words, if we see the family as purely a communication or meaning-making system, then we negate the impact that biological processes have on families. Genes, evolution, our physiological responses, our brains, our bodies, our emotions are all biological processes. If we are ignoring these processes, then we are overlooking factors that have given the family its autonomy and adaptability.

To illustrate what I mean, let's return to a Rosslenbroich quote from earlier. He wrote:

> On the one hand, there is the organism, and on the other hand is the environment. The organism – even in its simplest form – always establishes its life function together with the generation of a boundary and thus produces its 'being different' from the surrounding environment. To maintain this state, the organism not only needs regulatory and stabilizing functions on the one hand but needs to react appropriately to cope successfully with the environmental influences.

Let's edit some of the words in this quote to better illustrate the relationship between the family system and the social systems that create its environment:

> On the one hand, there is the [family system], and on the other hand is the [social system]. The [family system] – even in its simplest form – always establishes its life function together with the generation of a boundary and thus produces its 'being different' from the surrounding [social] environment. To maintain this state, the [family system]

not only needs regulatory and stabilizing functions on the one hand but needs to react appropriately to cope successfully with the [**social**] environmental influences.

The family system is different than the social system, but it must adapt to the social environmental influences to maintain its autonomy. Family systems today look different than family systems of 100 years ago, and very different than family systems of 1,000s of years ago. Part of the reason is because communication and conflicts of social systems have evolved over the years. If you go back and read "marriage advice" from the early 1900s, it is viewed as, at best, problematic, and, at worst, sexist and racist. And if there were marriage advice in 1000 BC, I'm sure it would have been even worse. The interactions that have occurred within the family system have adapted to social environmental influences.

The family system adapts, but it can also resist. The family system has been instrumental in changing the social systems. Often this resistance has come from those family systems that didn't benefit from the social environment. Though they were excluded from the power and resources, they demonstrated robustness to the social systems and created conflict that led to changes in the prevailing narratives about what a family is and who gets to be a part it. If marriage advice looks any better today than it did 100 or 1,000 years ago, it is because families that didn't have access to power fought for it and won.

It's important to point out that saying the family is a biological system isn't to imply that all of its members must be related – shared genes aren't required to create a family system. Families have and continue to be comprised of all sorts of people. Being a biological system just means that the system is autonomous and adaptable.

Family Systems Theory

I want to tie together the information we discussed in this chapter so far by providing a definition of family systems theory. This description is pulled from my previous book (Priest, 2021), but I want to include it to introduce some of the concepts that stem from the assumptions and definitions I've provided.

Family systems theory predicts and explains how people within a family interact, and how these interactions are different from outside the family. The family system is created by the genetic, individual, attachment, and triangulation systems and is shaped by the sociocultural system in which the family is embedded. Each of these systems are autonomous – they have processes that generate and maintain the system; and adaptable – they sense stimuli in the environment and within the family system to make reversible and irreversible changes based on the intensity of the stimulus. Autonomy and adaptation are created by at least three processes – threat response, belonging, and individuality. These processes, though unique, are interdependent, follow patterns or rules, and together create the unique interactions of the family system.

In my previous book, I aimed to provide convincing evidence for each of the statements in this paragraph. Here, however, I'm not going to go over that evidence again. I do want to talk about each of the statements in this description of family systems theory, but my goal for doing it this time around is different. I'm going to explain each of these sentences individually, so that I can provide the knowledge you'll need about family systems theory to make systemic diagnoses. Where it's applicable, I'll provide you with some concrete examples.

Family systems theory predicts and explains how people within a family interact, and how these interactions are different from outside the family.
For family systems theory to be an actual theory it needs predictive and explanatory power. If you can't predict and explain, you can't diagnose. What is family systems theory trying to predict and explain? Interactions. Interactions are what takes elements and makes them a system. But these interactions must be distinct from interactions that occur in other systems. For family systems theory to do its job, it has to explain how the interactions that occur in a family system are unique or distinct from interactions that occur in other systems.

Before we go any further, we do need to be clear on what constitutes an interaction. To do that, we first need to be clear about another word, *process*. If you notice, often these words get used interchangeably when talking about systems. But when we make systemic diagnoses, we are going to need to know about what in the family system constitutes an interaction and what constitutes a process. The difference between them is dependent on the system of interest. Let me explain that a bit more.

Suppose that you are observing a couple on a date at a restaurant. If the system that we are interested in is the couple system, the interactions of the couple system are what happens between them. If one person reaches out and touches the hand of the other person and the other person responds by pulling their hand back, that is an interaction. But that interaction is created by the processes that happened within each person. Within the person who reached their hand out, a multitude of other systems were interacting to get the person to feel the emotion, get up the courage, and then physically move their hand. For the other person to pull their hand away, systems within them had to sense the touch, interpret what it meant, generate a feeling of disgust, and then physically pull their hand away. Watching the couple, we were able to see the interaction – reaching out a hand and pulling out a hand. We aren't, however, seeing the processes that are happening within each of them.

If we change our system of interest to be just the individual who pulled back their hand, then we could examine the interactions that were going on inside of them – granted this might not be possible at a restaurant; we would need special equipment to analyze their brain and nervous system. That is why process and interaction get used interchangeably. One system's interactions are another system's processes. Often, we infer what the processes were that led to the interaction, even though we may not have directly observed them.

To predict and explain interactions in the family system, we are going to need to understand the processes that are happening within the other systems or elements that create the family system. If we are going to predict and explain interactions, we are going to need to know what processes spur on these interactions. That leads us to our next statement of the family systems theory description.

The family system is created by the genetic, individual, attachment, and triangulation systems and is shaped by the sociocultural system in which the family is embedded.

The family system isn't a system of isolation. It is a system that is created by interconnected systems. Though there are probably many more systems that create and shape the family system, for me, the evidence overwhelmingly points to the five systems I've listed in the statement earlier. To help me remember them – especially when making systemic diagnoses – I use the acronym GIAnTS. This acronym stands for the Genetic, Individual, Attachment, Triangulation, and Sociocultural. Each of these systems has elements, interactions, and purpose. Each of these systems can be seen as complete systems. But these systems create and shape the family system – they are the elements of the family system

I'm not going to detail all the research that connects each of these systems to the family system – I also did this in my previous work. Rather, I'm just going to give a quick overview of the important elements of each of these systems. The genetic system includes not only our genes but evolution by natural selection and the epigenome. These elements of the genetic system are the foundation of the family system and give rise to the individual system. The individual system is comprised of many systems – the cardiovascular system, the brain and nervous system, and many others. This system also includes the emotions, cognitions, and identities that arise from the nervous, cardiovascular, and other systems.

When two individuals form a relationship, this is the attachment system. The attachment system includes all the interactions that occur between two people, but also the processes that are happening in the genetic and individual systems. There are many combinations of attachment systems – two romantic partners, two parents, a parent and child, a grandparent and a grandchild. But these attachment systems don't exist in isolation. Individual systems are often never just a part of one attachment system. This is what gives rise to the triangulation system. An individual's attachment with one person is affected by and affects their attachment to another system. For example, two partners' attachment system is affected by the attachment they have to a parent, or to a child, or to a sibling, or to a grandparent.

The interactions and processes that happen in the attachment and triangulation system are what become the interactions or structure of the family system. These interactions and processes depend on the emotions, reactions, and genetic and epigenetic makeup of the individual systems of the family system.

The sociocultural system is the social system in which the family resides. This system includes not only systems that are communication and conflict based – like the law, politics, and religion – but environmental systems – like weather, climate, transportation, and infrastructure. The boundary between the genetic, individual, attachment, triangulation, and family systems is dynamic both across families and across time. The dynamic boundary between the family system and the sociocultural system is evident often in the language or communication that we make about families. The phrases father, son, brother, or uncle are not only markers of relationships but also markers of gender and power. Additionally, the same individual may inhabit different roles within the same family system across time. A son may become an uncle or father. A father may become a grandfather.

When creating systemic diagnosis based on family systems theory, it is important to remember the distinct attributes of the GIANTS systems but also to acknowledge the dynamic connections that exist between them.

Each of these systems are autonomous – they have processes that generate and maintain the system; and adaptable – they sense stimuli in the environment and within the family system to make reversible and irreversible changes based on the intensity of the stimulus.

When it comes to the biological systems that create the family system – each of them has the property of autonomy and adaptation. We have an abundance of research that shows that genetic, individual, and attachment systems have the property of autonomy and adaptation. We have less for the triangulation system. However, the research that does exist shows that the triangulation system also has processes that generate and maintain it and that it can adapt. We also have research that shows that the family system also has the properties of autonomy and adaptation.

These systems are often adapting to the social systems in which they reside. Though these social systems by their definition aren't biological systems, they do impact the biological processes of autonomy and adaptation. In other words, because of the communication and conflict that exist in social systems, family must adapt the autonomy generating processes to cater to the current social systems. Often, when families fail to adapt, the systems suffer. But remember, adapting in the biological sense doesn't mean just changing to the whim of the social system. Resilience and robustness are key adaptive processes.

Autonomy and adaptation are created by at least three processes – threat response, belonging, and individuality.

Up to this point, we've talked a lot about interactions and processes, but I want to take some time to talk about the interactions and processes that are the most important to the family system. These are the threat response, belonging, and individuality processes. Other processes can and do exist in the family, but these three processes are the core of the family system's autonomy and adaptability. Moreover, as I showed in my previous book, these three processes or interactions are backed by research. In other words, we have evidence of the threat response, belonging, and individuality processes occurring in the genetic, individual, attachment, triangulation, and family systems.

Because these processes are so important, I want to spend a bit of space in this chapter defining and describing them. Being able to recognize and diagnose these processes will be key to creating systemic diagnosis. Let's start by talking about the threat-response processes and interactions.

Threat-response processes include all the interactions that occur within systems that help us respond to changes – either within the system or the environment. We have lots of evidence to support the importance of threat-response processes. The fight, flight, or freeze response is an example of the threat-response processes. The signaling that occurs in the epigenome is another example. Our DNA doesn't change throughout our life, but the epigenome can respond to changes in our environment and affect the expression of genes. The attachment system is rooted in threat response processes; as is the triangulation system. If we are separated from an attachment figure, our threat-response processes are activated to motivate us to reconnect. If we can't reconnect, we may bring in another person to stand in place or replace the lost connection.

Threat-response processes motivate us to respond to change. Change within the system or in the environment provokes a reaction in the system – this reaction is felt as stress or anxiety. The system responds to the change and accompanying stress by adapting. This can include getting spatial separation from the change; being more robust or more flexible; internalizing the change; or by expanding the system. The activation of threat-response processes can create reversible and irreversible changes in a system. For example, if the system expands, the new person added to the system may stick around forever, or they may just be present for a short time. The system may develop a new level of flexibility just until the change passes, or the increased flexibility may be the new state of the system.

Threat-response processes are key to a system's autonomy. If systems don't have threat-response processes, they can't adapt. If they can't adapt, they lose their autonomy. That is why we often think of threat-response processes being connected to survival. All systems, not just the family system or the systems that create the family system, have threat-response processes. It could be argued that threat-response processes are the key to system generation and perpetuation.

But there are two other processes of the family system that build on and respond to the threat response processes. These are the belonging and individuality processes. The belonging processes include all the interactions that maintain interrelations between elements in a system. The individual processes include all the interactions that maintain the autonomy of elements within a system.

For a system to maintain autonomy it must have interrelations – elements must be connected. The belonging process of the family system is what maintains the connections between elements. The belonging processes can include feelings of love, or interactions that promote bonding and intimacy. It can also include interactions that try to establish control or power, or coerce connection. This can include intensely monitoring someone's behavior within other systems or rigid family rules that try to force the family to stay together. Belonging processes are any interactions that are the impetus for maintaining the system's autonomy. They keep the system together and keep the system going.

For a system to maintain autonomy it must also have discrete elements. Each discrete element contributes to the distinct interactions that occur within the system. If the elements fuse together the system can't survive. The individuality processes of the family system are what maintains the elements' autonomy. Elements of a system are also systems themselves – individuals that are the elements of the family system are also autonomous systems. If the elements of a system lose their autonomy, then the autonomy of the larger system that the element is embedded in may also lose its autonomy. In the family system examples of individuality processes can include pushing back against expectations, carving out a unique identity, or being rebellious. It can also be pursuing goals or dreams, or the development of skills or abilities. individuality processes are any interactions that are the impetus for an element in a system to maintain autonomy. They keep the elements discrete.

> These processes, though unique, are interdependent, follow patterns or rules, and together create the unique interactions of the family system.

The threat response, belonging, and individuality processes are unique, but in the family system they are interdependent. They are key to understanding the interactive and constitutive dimensions of adaptation of the family system. Remember, the interactive dimension of autonomy is considered with factors that reduce (or potentially increase) the effect, influence, or power that the environment has on the system. The constitutive dimension concerns the enhancement of the interactions or processes that provide stability and flexibility for the system.

If there is a change in the family system or in their environment, the threat-response processes are engaged. The engagement of the threat-response processes often results in the engagement of the belonging or individuality processes. If the family is under threat from the loss of a job, the family may intensify the belonging process to weather that change in the environment. They may show more support to the family member who lost the job or they may pool their resources. On the other hand the family could respond by intensifying the individuality processes. The other family members may start looking for other jobs or take on additional responsibilities to help the family weather the change. They also may do both.

Changes in the environment may engage the threat-response process, leading to the intensification of the belonging or individuality processes, but the intensification of the belonging or individuality processes can also engage the threat-response processes. If the belonging processes in a family system are too intense, they may trigger the threat-response processes in one or more elements of a system. The triggering of the threat-response process would lead to the intensification of the individuality process of the elements that were triggered. This can be seen in families where a child may have disordered eating. The interactions of the belonging processes may be so intense that the child's threat-response processes are activated, leading to the intensification of the child's individuality processes. The intensification of the individuality processes may manifest as restricting – giving the child at least some sense of control of themselves.

The interdependence of these processes can look different across different elements of the family system. Let's take for example an attachment system that includes two romantic partners. If these two partners are going on a date, this is an interaction that serves to strengthen the belonging processes of this system. At the same time this is also an individuality process – as the couple is showing the other attachment systems in the family system that this interaction is something that the partner attachment system does that makes it distinct from the other attachment systems. In other words, the belonging process of an attachment system may be viewed as an individuality process in the broader family system.

From Theory to Therapy Room

This chapter has introduced lots of concepts – elements; process; interactions; GIANTS, the constitutive, interactive, and historical dimensions;

communication; conflict; and, of course, autonomy and adaptation. While process and interactions, communication and conflict, are terms that family therapists use frequently, the others are not. But I want to use words that family therapists are familiar with as we transition from theory to therapy room. If you recall in Chapter 3, I argued that if we don't have a deep knowledge of theory, we could create poor diagnoses, which could result in bad interventions. Because of that, I wanted to use the language that is found in biological and social systems theories to introduce these concepts. But, I also understand that to make this portable to the therapy room, we need to not only ground it in evidence-based theory, but also make it accessible. So, I want to propose a change in terms to two of the dimensions of adaptation.

If you look at the constitutive dimension, it's synonymous with what family systems theory would call "structure." I haven't used this word earlier on, because "structure" in family therapy can sometimes mean many different things. But when using family systems theory, "structure" isn't about what the family is – single-parent family, multigenerational family – nor is it necessarily about hierarchy – who has power or who is more important. In family systems theory, "structure" is a description of the intrinsic systemic interactions or processes that provide stability and flexibility for the family system. These interactions may create a hierarchy but the hierarchy itself isn't a structure. The structure of a family system is about the interactions of the elements of the system. In other words, the structure of the family is a description of the constitutive dimension of their system.

If you look at the properties of the interactive dimension, family therapists would typically refer to this as a boundary. I've stayed away from this word so far, because this word has been co-opted by social media influencers and others to just mean to "say no" to someone who asks you for something. But if we are using family systems theory the word "boundary" has a more complex meaning. It is how the structure of the family system shifts interactions to increase or decrease the influence of the environment on the family system. To me that is much different than just "saying no." If we think about boundaries as shifting interactions and structures to regulate the influence of the environment, we get a much richer and more useful definition of boundaries. When we describe a family's boundaries, we are describing the interactive dimension of their system.

Going forward, I'm going to use the words "structure" and "boundary" in place of "constitutive dimension" and "interactive dimension." But every time I do, I want you to think about how these words used in family systems theory are different from their more colloquial usage. I'm still going to use historical dimension, but I'll use it interchangeably with development and family of origin – words that therapists are also familiar with. The history of the system includes the elements and inter-actions that were previously in the system and the developmental stage or trajectory of the system currently.

As you'll see in the next chapter, the process of systemic diagnosis – based in family systems theory – results in a clear description of the history, structure, and boundaries of a family system. To get a clear description of family system, we are going to need to know what elements, pur-poses, interactions, and contexts (the communication and conflict of the social system) are shaping the structure and boundaries of the system. That is what Chapter 5 is all about. As you'll see, a systemic diagnosis isn't checking to see whether a family has a list of symptoms that means they qualify for a certain diagnosis; rather, using family systems theory, therapists can create clear, meaningful descriptions of the system. These descriptions or diagnoses set them up to intervene effectively. But before we go there, I've again summarized the main arguments and ideas of this chapter next.

Recap: Main Ideas and Arguments

1. **For decades, family therapists have been unable to clearly define or describe family systems theory.** Instead of being a theory, family systems theory has really become more of a col-lection of vague ideas. Some have argued, with good evidence, that Bowen's family systems theory contains a clear set of test-able hypotheses. However, the assumptions of Bowen's theory are built on ideas that in some instances have been disproven or made obsolete by new research.

2. **Family therapists also aren't always clear on how to define "system."** A system has three components – elements, interac-tions, and purpose. Elements are the things that interact, and the interactions of the elements are what describe its purpose.

3. **The family system is a biological system embedded in social systems.** Biological systems are autonomous – they have pro-cesses that generate and maintain the system – and adaptable – they make reversible and irreversible changes based on their internal state and their environment. Social systems are used to secure power and access to resources. The elements of social systems are communication and conflict.

4. **Family systems theory predicts and explains how people within a family interact.** The family system is created by the genetic,

individual, attachment, and triangulation systems. Each of these systems is autonomous and adaptable.

5. **Autonomy and adaptation in a family system are generated and maintained by the threat-response, belonging, and individuality processes.** Threat-response processes include all the interactions of elements in a system that respond to change. The belonging processes are any interactions that are the impetus for keeping the elements of a system together. Individuality processes are any interactions that maintain the discreetness of the elements of a system.

Chapter 5

Systemic Diagnosis

If you are currently in a family therapy training program, or if you have graduated from one, you probably have done a case conceptualization for a practicum class. In my experience, the way this is done varies widely but there have been those who have pushed to create guidelines for the way that case conceptualization could be done. One of those who have written extensively about case conceptualization is Len Sperry. Sperry (2005) defines conceptualization as:

> a method and process of summarizing seemingly diverse case information into a brief, coherent statement or "map" that elucidates that client's basic patterns of behavior. The purpose of a well-articulated case conceptualization is to better understand and more effectively treat a client or client-system, namely the couple or family. In short, a case conceptualization is a clinician's 'theory' of a particular case.

In that same article, Sperry provides examples of how he argues that case conceptualization should be done. He recommends that case conceptualization should include a diagnostic formation (based on the DSM), and clinical formation, and a treatment formation.

Similarly, in 2016, Michael Reiter wrote an article on case conceptualization arguing that they included "a theory of the problem and a theory of the problem resolution" and added that a case can be conceptualized from any "theoretical model." For example, Reiter provides what he calls the "6 Ps" of case conceptualization from a Structural Family Therapy lens – problem, process, pattern, proximity, power, and possibilities.

While I think that both Sperry and Reiter make good points, they are also making a big mistake: conflating theory, diagnosis, and intervention. Sperry talks about creating a map that talks about the client's basic patterns of behavior. But without theory, how do we know what patterns are important and what patterns are not? Reiter talks about the

DOI: 10.4324/9781003295907-7

conceptualization of the problem and the conceptualization of problem resolution. But without theory, how do we know what constitutes a problem and what constitutes the resolution of the problem?

It also seems that Reiter and, to a lesser extent, Sperry are using interventions to conceptualize cases. If you are using Structural Family Therapy to conceptualize a case, your conceptualization isn't being circumscribed by theory but by intervention. That could result in missing really important information about the family. If you are using intervention to conceptualize, you can only conceptualize the factors where intervention is possible. I would argue that this would limit the possibilities that Reiter argues for.

Since these models of case conceptualization are not grounded in theory but by intervention, it's not always clear what you are looking for, or why you are looking for it. Take two of Reiter's "Ps" – process and pattern. For him a process is "the idiosyncratic way in which people come together at a specific point in time." And pattern is "family processes that occur over time." In writing about them, he writes about things we covered in Chapter 4 – interactions, boundaries, and adaptation.

But because they aren't rooted in theory, the definitions he provides are at best confusing and at worst contradictory. If a process is idiosyncratic or unique to a certain time point, at what point does it stop being idiosyncratic enough to be a pattern? If the process is just at a certain time point, if it continues to happen at other time points is it not a process? Is it now just a pattern? What's more, these definitions don't tell you which processes or patterns are important, or which aren't. There also isn't any explanation or hypotheses about why processes or patterns occur.

If you dive a bit deeper into Sperry's and Reiter's writings, you'll notice that the case examples they provide aren't really about conceptualization or diagnosis, but more about intervention. Reiter's case examples explain what the therapist does to intervene. He talks more about enactments, asking questions that could shift patterns, than he does describe the history, structure, and boundaries of the system. Don't get me wrong, what Reiter is doing I think is good therapy – his interventions seem solid. It's just disconnected from what he and Sperry write about the goal of case conceptualization.

Now, you could be reading this and be thinking, "Isn't this just semantics? Does it really matter if we are providing a systemic diagnosis or a case conceptualization? Aren't they just the same thing using different words?" Or you may be thinking, "Doth Jacob protest too much? Isn't he trying to exacerbate differences that really aren't that different? Is he just defensive that somebody has already beat him to his idea?"

I think those are fair questions to ask. So, before I present the procedures of systemic diagnosis, I want to make a case as to why I see them as different.

Theory-Driven Diagnosis

In Chapter 3, I argued that the role of theory in family therapy was to circumscribe possible explanations and set the parameters of diagnosis. You can't diagnose something that your theory doesn't hold in the realm of possibility. If your diagnosis isn't explicitly tied to theory, then you could have limitless possibilities. Your diagnosis could also be tied to bad theory. If your theory is that all problems in families are a result of Angen abduction, and you diagnose a family with "Angen abduction syndrome," your intervention might be creating shelters so that families don't get abducted. My guess is that if you said this to most families, they'd probably find a different therapist.

Good theory provides an evidence-based explanation for the current context. It provides limits on what is possible, and a rationale for why this is the case. It can tell you what is important, and what is not. It can explain why something is important and predict what will happen given the current state. Good theory can also be challenged and falsified – because good theory is built on assumptions and hypotheses. Those assumptions and hypotheses can be tested. If evidence doesn't support the assumptions and hypotheses, then they need to be changed or discarded.

Case conceptualization as currently practiced and described by Sperry and Reiter is either atheoretical or intervention based. Without a theory driving the diagnosis or conceptualization, therapists are then creating their own "theories." These theories are typically ad hoc explanations of what they saw. Instead of setting parameters that help therapists focus on what is important, these ad hoc explanations can be more about what the therapist thinks they can do to intervene. The thought processes is, "I can do an enactment here, so that means that this must be an important pattern." This atheoretical, intervention-driven approach may make the therapist seem like they know what's going on, but they may in fact be missing important information because they are so focused on doing.

Systemic diagnosis is theory driven. It is rooted in family systems theory. Family systems theory is an evidence-based theory, built on the assumption that the family is a biological system embedded in a social environment. It hypothesized that the family is an autonomous and adaptable system. These assumptions and hypotheses limit possible explanations making it possible for the therapist to know what is important to assess and what is not. Unlike the intervention-driven process of case conceptualization, systemic diagnosis uses theory and diagnosis to decide how an intervention should occur.

Problems Versus Autonomy and Adaptation

Case conceptualization is about problems. Case conceptualization is about creating an ad hoc theory of the problem that is predetermined by the intervention framework the therapist has already chosen. This is evident in some therapists labeling themselves a "Structural Family Therapist," or a "Narrative Therapist," or a "Solution-Focused Therapist." The therapist already has chosen the framework for intervention and is going to describe the problem in a way that they feel comfortable intervening.

Systemic diagnosis is about observing and gathering information about the system that describes its history, structure, and boundaries. If you remember in Chapter 4, structure is the constitutive dimension of autonomy and adaptation, and boundaries are the interactive dimension of autonomy and adaptation. Because systemic diagnosis is theory driven, problems aren't limited based on what the therapist feels comfortable intervening in, but the information about the autonomous and adaptive state of the system. Family systems theory provides an explanation and prediction around "problems." In family systems theory a "problem" isn't what the family wants fixed, it is telling you about the system's history, structure, and boundaries.

Granted, in some frameworks of case conceptualization, the creators of the framework would argue that the problem is also information about what is going on in the system. But because the case conceptualization is atheoretical or intervention driven, the information is used in a very different way. The information about the problem is used only to remove the problem. This is assuming that the problem can be fixed and that the preordained intervention that is conceptualizing the problem is the remedy.

However, family systems theory and systemic diagnosis make no such assumption about problems. In fact, you'll notice that in Chapter 4, the discussion of problems was almost nonexistent. That is because problems are part of the autonomy and adaptive functions of the system. In many instances they are described as problems because what is occurring in the system is trying to adapt to the messages that are dominant in the social environment. If the "problem" is too much anxiety, or a poorly behaved kid those definitions are telling you about the interactive dimension or boundaries of the system with the social environment.

Biological systems are not intrinsically social – they are autonomous. They have processes and interactions that generate and sustain the system. The family as a biological system is adapting their processes and interactions to the social and physical environment that it is embedded in and to the elements that construct the system. These adaptations are not problems, nor are they bad. They just are. They may be stressing the system, they may seem self-destructive, but they are just adaptations that are increasing or decreasing the autonomy of the system.

This also means that in family systems theory and systemic diagnosis not everything can be "solved." Genetic issues that structure an individual's autonomy often can't be "fixed." And in some cases, trying to fix it says more about the social messages of the environment than the individual or family system. People who are neurodivergent are often given therapy to "fix" their "problematic" social interactions, but these social interactions aren't "problems." Rather the "problems" that we assign to neurodivergent people reflect a social system that so inflexibly defines what is acceptable and what is not.

A systemic diagnosis details the autonomous and adaptive state of the system – it doesn't tell us what the problem is or how it is to be resolved. By not defining the problem as the problem, systemic diagnosis in fact gives the therapist more ways to intervene. If the "problem" is narrowly defined by the potential interventions, the options are reduced. If the autonomous and adaptive state of the system is well understood, a therapist then has multiple avenues to accelerate or decelerate adaptive trends, structure interactions, or renegotiate the influence that the environment has on the system.

The only "goal" or purpose that a system has is to maintain its autonomy – it does this by adapting its structure and boundaries based upon its history and the social environment. A systemic diagnosis doesn't give us the path to fix the problem, because systems aren't concerned with problems. Rather, systemic diagnosis describes the current state of the system and makes predictions, based on family systems theory, about the trajectory of the system.

Changing Autonomy

This isn't to say that family systems theory doesn't have anything to say about what contributes to a system maintaining its autonomy. Biological systems can change their autonomy – remember Rosslenbroich defined changes in autonomy as adaptation. Biological systems can increase their autonomy or lose their autonomy – some biological systems have been extinct for millennia. Family systems can and do change their autonomy. But the reasoning that family systems theory provides for this change is vastly different from an intervention, problem-focused, atheoretical case conceptualization.

In family systems theory, systems have adaptive trajectories. These trajectories are shaped by the history, structures, and boundaries of the system. Because each system has unique elements and interactions, the trajectories are never the same. But I want to talk briefly about two broad classes of trajectories – thriving trajectories and disintegrating trajectories. We'll talk much more about these trajectories in Chapter 12. Again, systems shouldn't be classified as one or the other – trajectories can shift. But let's talk about both types of trajectories.

Systems on thriving trajectories are flexible and robust. When structural or environmental pressures are exacerbated beyond the typical homeostasis of the system, thriving systems adjust to reduce the pressure – sometimes these adjustments are permanent and sometimes they occur only for a short period of time. But systems with thriving trajectories don't just adapt by adjusting, they also adapt by being robust. These systems will use structural interactions to push back against pressure from the environment. They slow the pace of adaptation to not lose their constitutive integrity. Flexibility and robustness in systems with thriving trajectories can be responsive to the environment and to structural interactions. Flexibility and robustness work together to allow the system to adapt across time without consistently overburdening threat-response, belonging, and individuality processes. While these processes can be stressed in order to create the necessary changes, one process isn't abandoned in favor of another.

This isn't to say that thriving systems don't have friction – any adaptation that is made by the structure or boundary of a system will stress the system. But systems on thriving trajectories use this friction to maintain or increase their autonomy. The friction that results in changing interactions and boundaries, while creating discomfort, doesn't create the toxicity that leads to the breakdown of the system.

Instead of being flexible or robust, systems on disintegrating trajectories are typically one or the other, or are too much of both. If a system is on a pathway to disintegration, it may be too flexible – reacting strongly to any pressure from the structure or environment. It may make changes quickly that quell short-term stress but create unsustainable interactions or an unsustainable boundary with the environment. A system on a disintegrating trajectory may be too rigid. Structural, developmental, or environmental pressures may necessitate adaptation, but the system refuses to or can't adapt. The system may get stuck, or it may refuse to take in new information from the environment, but its inability to adapt weakens the system's structural and interactive integrity, leaving it in danger of disintegration.

It should be noted, however, that many systems that seem to be on a disintegrating trajectory, are in fact thriving systems that are in toxic environments. A system may be able to adapt well, but if the social and environmental system that the family system is embedded in is so toxic to the elements and interactions of the system, regardless of how well the system is able to adapt, it may not be enough. Many family systems are under threat of disintegration not because of poor interactions or boundaries, but because the social and environmental system they inhabit is destructive.

Also, I want to point out that when it comes to family system trajectories, they are disintegrating trajectories not disintegrated systems. Because of our cognitive and emotional capabilities, we still have interactions with family members even if that family member is cutoff or deceased. While some family systems may fully disintegrate, most will just continue a disintegrating trajectory. What's more, depending on the time when you encounter a family system, they may seem to be either a thriving or disintegrating system. However, systems can change trajectories. Things in the system and in the social environment can and do occur that can lead a system to be on different trajectories and different points.

Case conceptualization assumes that once the problem is solved therapy can end. If the clients have met their goals, because of the intervention that therapist used, the family will now be in a new state of homeostasis that is healthy functioning. But family systems theory makes no such assumption. Instead of problem solving, diagnosis and intervention in family systems theory is about facilitating adaptations that are both flexible and robust. It is about understanding the historical and current structure and boundaries of a family system to help alter the trajectory.

I'm hoping that you are at least somewhat convinced that systemic diagnosis is different from the way family therapists talk and teach about case conceptualization. To really make that decision, I'd recommend reading the work not only of Sperry and Reiter, but also others like Diane Gehart. If you examine their work, you may conclude, like I did, that case conceptualization is atheoretical and intervention driven, but you may not. Either way, I'm going to move on to describing and explaining how to diagnose a family system based on family systems theory. I'm hoping that even if you're not convinced, you'll critically examine this process and create something even better.

Diagnosing the Family System

Systemic diagnosis isn't case conceptualization; it isn't relational diagnosis; nor is it diagnosis based on the DSM. Systemic diagnosis is a description and explanation of the history, structure, and boundaries of a family system. Systemic diagnosis uses family systems theory to gather relevant information about a system and use this information to provide an account of the state of the system. This account set the stage for the potential avenues of intervention. The procedures of systemic diagnosis aren't new – like other types of diagnosis it's about gathering information and creating a diagnosis. What is different is what information is deemed important. In systemic diagnosis we gather information about four things – elements, purpose, interactions, and context. We use this information to create a systemic diagnosis – a statement of the history, structure, and boundaries of a system.

While I'm hoping the connection between systemic diagnosis and family systems theory is clear, I want to take just a little bit of space to make those connections explicit. The family is an autonomous system. It has elements that interact, and these interactions generate and maintain the system – giving the system its purpose or function. These interactions represent the constitutive dimension or structure of the family system. To describe and explain a family system's structure, we must have information about the elements, purpose, and interactions of the system. The family is also an adaptable system. The structure of the family system must respond to pressures from inside and outside the system. This is done by changing the structure to reshape the influence the environment has on the system – this is known as the interactive dimension or boundary of a family system. To describe and explain a family system's boundary, we need to know about the current and historical context of the family, and how this context shaped and is shaping the structure of the family.

Later, I'm going to walk through examples of the systemic diagnosis process. I'll give examples of questions that therapists can use to gather information about the element, purpose, interactions, and context of a system. I'll demonstrate how to take this information and create a description of the history, structure, and boundaries of a system. But before we do that, I think it's important to explain what exactly we are assessing when gathering information about the element, purpose, interactions, and context of a system; and the rationale for doing so. Gathering information about these factors of a family system allows us to answer the questions "who, where, how, and why?" Answering these questions, and formulating a diagnosis creates a platform for effective intervention.

Elements

To create a systemic diagnosis, we must know what elements are in a family system. We can't have a system without elements. If you remember from Chapter 4, elements are anything that interacts with another thing. When diagnosing a family system, there are three key elements we need to identify – the individual systems, the attachment systems, and the triangulation systems. Often when we think about the elements of the family system, we are just thinking about the individual people. But individuals are just one set of elements. Attachment systems interact and overlap with other attachment systems – so attachment systems are elements. Triangulation systems interact and overlap with other attachment and triangulation systems – so they are also elements.

It's important to note, however, that when identifying elements, we are probably not going to be able to keep all of them in mind. Let's say, for example, that there are six individuals in a family system. In addition to these six elements, there are potentially ten attachment systems, creating 16 elements. If you add on the potential number of triangles – another ten elements, you have 26 elements. If you are looking at a family system with ten individuals, there is the potential to have 175 elements. When identifying elements, it's important to keep in mind the complexity, that complexity can be useful when intervening. However, if the goal is to make sure you are identifying all the potential elements of a family system with each client you work with, you'll never be able move beyond identifying elements.

What's more, you'll remember in the previous chapter I talked about the systems that create the family system – or the elements of a family system. I used the acronym GIANTS – this stood for Genetic, Individual, Attachment, Triangulation, Sociocultural systems. You'll notice that in gathering information to create a systemic diagnosis, I'm not focusing on the genetic system (we'll focus on the Sociocultural system in the "context" section). This isn't because I don't think that the genetic system is important. It's because the current ability to assess the genetic system isn't something that can be used in a therapy room – at least not yet. There are many companies that are creating genetic profiles based on samples that people send to them (e.g., 23andMe, Ancestry.com) but at the time of this writing, family therapists aren't trained to make genetic assessments, and these tools aren't being used to create assessment in therapy. Given the explosion of research around genes and the genome, it may be that eventually family therapists will be trained to use tools to assess the impact of genetics on the structure and boundaries of the family system. But because it isn't currently available, we won't be talking about how to assess the genetic system.

Identifying individual elements and attachment elements is relatively straightforward – it's embedded in our language. If I say, "Scott is my father," I'm identifying an individual element, me (Jacob) and Scott, and an attachment relationship, father-son. If I say, "Birdie is my daughter," or "Birdie is Scott's granddaughter," I'm identifying individual elements – me (Jacob), Birdie, and Scott, and three attachment elements – father-daughter, grandfather-granddaughter, and father-son. While this language or communication describes the relationships, the label given to these individual elements and their attachment systems also send messages about power in these relationship – we'll talk more about that in the "context" section.

Identifying triangles sometimes isn't as straightforward – but if you look a bit more carefully at the language, we do describe triangles all the time. For example, if you are out to lunch with your spouse and your child, and you run into a work friend who hasn't met them before, you'll probably introduce them by saying, "Work friend, this is my wife, Chelsea, and our daughter, Birdie." You've described individual elements, and attachment elements, but you've also described a triangle. My wife, Chelsea, and me (Jacob), are an attachment element, so is Chelsea and Birdie, and so is Birdie and me. Three attachment elements make a triangle. If I was out to lunch with my wife and both kids and ran into a work friend, and said, "Work friend, this is my wife, Chelsea, my son, Keenan, and our daughter, Birdie," I would be describing four triangles – Jacob-Chelsea-Keenan; Jacob-Chelsea-Birdie; Jacob-Keenan-Birdie; Chelsea-Keenan-Birdie.

Assessing the element of the system answers the important question, "who?" In other words, it tells us who are the people who are interacting with each other; who are the elements that create attachment systems; who are in the attachment systems that create the triangles. If we are going to create a systemic diagnosis, we need to know who the elements of the system are.

Purpose

Once we identify the elements of a system, we need a way to focus on what is important and what isn't. We do this through assessing the purpose of a system. When assessing a family system, it may seem that there are multiple purposes. Families may come to therapy with multiple "goals." But since family systems theory assumes that the family is a biological system, it only has one purpose – maintaining autonomy. The reason for the seemingly multiple purposes is that the family system is created by elements that are also systems – the individual, attachment, and triangulation systems. These systems all want to maintain their autonomy – and sometimes the interactions that are occurring within each of these systems may threaten the autonomy of one or more other systems.

To create a systemic diagnosis, we are going to need to track the interactions of the family system, and the interactions of the elements that create it. But as we talked about, systems are created by multiple elements – creating dozens or hundreds of interactions. This makes it nearly impossible to track all the interactions that are occurring in the system. To make a meaningful diagnosis, we need a way to reduce the number of interactions that we are assessing. To do this, we assess where the elements seem to be competing for autonomy.

Because each element of the family system strives to maintain itself, it must justify the interactions that occur in multiple systems. This is typically done through the stories and narratives that are shared with the therapist. Many times, these narratives and stories get construed as the purpose or problem of the system. However, this isn't the case. Rather, the narratives and stories can be used to identify locations of competing autonomy. For example, triangulation systems are built on attachment systems. What may serve to sustain the autonomy of one or two attachment systems may be a threat to the autonomy of the triangle. The purpose of each attachment system to generate and maintain itself is going to structure the interactions of the triangulation system. These interactions get translated and told in therapy as stories and narratives.

If a family comes to therapy because there is one child who is the problem, this narrative is useful not to gather information about the problematic child, but rather because it helps the therapist narrow down which elements need their interactions assessed. In other words, it's likely that the attachment and triangulation systems that this child inhabits are where the interactions that threaten or are viewed as a threat to the autonomy of other elements are occurring. The narratives that the family shares about the problematic child aren't necessarily "true," rather they are manifestations where elements have competing autonomy. Remember autonomy is the interactions that serve to generate and maintain the system. Elements of the family system have competing autonomy when interactions push for adaptations that threaten the current autonomy of other elements. Getting the family to share these narratives is important to create a systemic diagnosis, not so that the therapist will believe the narrative, but rather to help the therapist identify where the therapist should focus their attention.

Therapists often use the phrase "process over content" to help them not to get caught up in the narratives a family brings. But I think that this misses an important step. We need to focus on purpose, not just process and content. If we focus on process or interactions without thinking about purpose, we may inadvertently have too narrow of a focus. For example, the narrative that one child is the problem may lead a therapist to focus on the process of just one attachment system – diagnosing this system as where the intervention needs to occur. However, focusing on just one attachment system obscures that there are multiple attachment systems that create multiple triangles in the family system. If we diagnose and just intervene on one attachment system, we may create a pattern of interaction that threatens the autonomy of a triangle. To create a systemic diagnosis, we use content to find competing purposes that show us where to assess the process.

Assessing the purpose or competing purposes of a system helps the therapist strike a balance between focusing too broadly or to narrowly in the family system. Assessing all the elements and interactions would be nearly impossible but focusing too narrowly on one element or one system may create new points of competing purposes – leading interventions to fall flat. If we identify the places where competing purposes exist in a system, it helps us focus our assessment on multiple systems. Assessing the purpose or competing purposes of the system answers "where" questions. It tells us where to look and what to look for. By assessing the purpose, we can find the signal in the noise – we can focus on certain elements and systems and the interactions that are creating "the problem."

Interactions

Once we've identified the elements of the family system, and the elements where competition for autonomy occurs, we can begin to assess the interactions of the system. Tracking interactions is quite common in family therapy, but when creating a systemic diagnosis, we aren't just tracking who does what, we are trying to identify the rules of the interactions. If the purpose of the elements of the system is to maintain their autonomy, and the "problems" that families bring to therapy are instances where there is competition of purpose, the rules of the interactions are how the family tries to maintain autonomy.

If you remember, in the previous chapter, I talked about the difference between processes and interactions. Put succinctly: one system's interactions are another system's processes. Or put another way, processes of individual systems create the interactions of attachment systems; processes of attachment systems create the interactions of triangulation systems; and the processes of individual, attachment, and triangulation systems are the interactions of the family systems.

When assessing the processes and interactions of a family system, we are focused on three of them – threat-response, belonging, and individuality. If you remember, threat-response processes motivate us to respond to change, threats, or new information within the system or in the environment. Belonging processes are interactions that maintain connections between elements. Individual processes are interactions that help maintain the autonomy of the elements in the system. These are the processes and interactions that give the family system its autonomy. Without these interactions, the family system isn't a system.

Interactions are what give a system its autonomy – interactions generate and maintain the system. To do this, interactions have rules or patterns that they follow. These rules or patterns tell the elements how to react when something threatens the autonomy of the system or elements within the system. When looking to identify the rules of the interactions, it's important to keep in mind that threat-response, belonging, and individuality processes are interdependent. Often a rule that a system follows is based on more than one of these processes.

The rules of a system are not like the rules of a classroom. Classroom rules are linear – if you talk out of turn you get a demerit. The rules of the system are what the system does (the interactions that happen) to generate and maintain itself; what it does when it feels its autonomy is threatened; what it does when it is trying to increase its autonomy; or what it does when it is making reversible or irreversible changes to respond to the environment. Rules of a family system occur within and between the multiple elements in the system – the processes that each element takes to complete these rules may be different – some may have more belonging processes, others may have more individuality processes – but the rule spans the systems. In family systems theory, rules tend to fall into a few domains. Family systems create rules around homeostasis – how the system tries to keep things the same; there are rules around flexibility – how the system responds to acute and chronic changes; there are rules around how the system separates itself from its environment. The homeostasis and flexibility rules are rules about the constitutive dimension or structure of the system. Separation from the environment rules are about the interactive dimension or boundary of the system.

Homeostasis is what establishes and enhances internal functioning. Homeostatic rules use threat-response, belonging, and individual interactions to try and regulate stability or maintain a constant internal environment. Systems use homeostatic rules to set the range of variation or influence that elements or the environment can have. If the environment or the elements exceed the range, the homeostatic rules activate the interactions to bring it back into that range. Most family systems will have homeostatic rules. While the interactions that enforce these rules are different, the existence of the rules is often key to the system's autonomy.

Flexibility rules are about reversible and irreversible changes to interactions. Flexibility reflects a system's ability to generate functional answers to conditions or changes in the environment. These rules reflect how a system adapts during a crisis or how a system changes over time. Flexibility rules specify what types of changes can happen in the threat-response, individuality, and belonging processes and what types cannot. Flexibility rules aim to help the system increase or maintain its autonomy by giving it some degree of freedom in the interactions of the system.

The rules about separation from the environment specify how a system keeps the environment outside of the system. Without these rules, the environment may overwhelm the system, resulting in the system losing its autonomy. However, the system can never be fully differentiated from its environment, so separation rules also regulate exchanges with the environment. The threat-response, individuality, and belonging processes that occur in the elements of a system help the system stay connected to the environment without being overwhelmed by it.

The rules of interactions of a system are oftentimes most assessable during stress. When a system is not under stress, or the interactions of the elements in a system aren't creating competition for autonomy, the rules are sometimes hard to identify – they are there, but they seem to fade into the background. When under stress, or when the rules no longer fit the development of the elements or the current environment, this is when they can be more readily assessed.

Rules of interaction of a system answer the question "how?" These rules tell us how the system has maintained its autonomy over time and how it is trying to maintain its autonomy now. It tells us the patterns or steps that the elements of the family system take when interacting with each other and when interacting with the environment. Assessing the rules of interactions that a system has created is key to creating a systemic diagnosis.

Context

Typically, when creating a diagnosis, we tend not to assess much beyond the system of interest – we don't assess the environment that the system is embedded in. When a psychiatrist is assessing whether a patient meets DSM-5 criteria for depression, they aren't typically asking about the environment – sociocultural or physical – in which the patient resides. The diagnostic criteria don't require that. However, when creating a systemic diagnosis, understanding the environment that the system is embedded in is key to formulating a diagnosis. The reason for the presence or absence of certain elements, locations of competing autonomy, and the rules of interactions of the system are dependent on the environmental context. You can't understand the system without understanding its environment.

The context or environment of the system is its developmental niche (Oyama, 2000). The system develops in the environment its embedded and that environment shaped and molds the interactions of the system. The present context of the system is dependent on the history of the system. The historical dimension of the system details how the system developed its rules of interaction and how those have changed in response to internal and environmental pressures. It is a history of how the system has negotiated its interactions in the environment and how these negotiations have shifted the boundary between the family and the environment. The context also described the present system-environment relationship and how this relationship creates competition of purpose between elements of the system. Context is both the history and the present of how a system has maintained and is maintaining its autonomy in the changing environment.

To create a systemic diagnosis, a therapist must be well versed in the past and present context of the system. Without understanding the historical and current developmental context of the system, the explanation of elements, purpose, and interaction is incomplete. The context of a family system is built by the social systems and the physical space where the family resides. If you remember from Chapter 4, a social system is about the cultural narratives that aim to justify the current allocation of resources. These narratives reflect those in power and the stories that are used to justify the current power hierarchy. Often these social systems shape the physical space in which a family system resides. If social systems try and justify current resource allocation, then this is often reflected in the physical space. These two factors – the social systems and the physical space – are the environment that the family must navigate. The interactions that are occurring within the family system reflect how the family navigate their context.

The context of a family system is not only reflected in the interactions but also in the elements themselves. In many social systems, the elements are given identity markers by the social system that serve to conscript the "acceptable" interactions of a given element. For example, in many social systems, cisgender men are given the identity marker of "husband" and "father" and cisgender women are given the identity marker of "wife" and "mother." These identity markers are social communications that often serve to reinforce the current power hierarchy. As a father, the amount of effort I must put in to been seen as a "super dad" is much less than what my wife must put in to just be a "regular mom." Her identity marker as a mother conscript her into certain interactions that she is not rewarded for by the power hierarchy, whereas when I do the same task, the social system rewards me by telling me how great I am. Our interactions in our marriage and as parents are conscripted by the social systems we inhabit.

But this doesn't only happen for individual elements, but attachment elements and triangulation elements also are given identity markers. In almost every culture the attachment element "marriage" comes with conscripted processes. Who can do what, how they do it, and when all exist prior to an actual marriage. In other words, before the marriage begins, the individual elements within the marriage have been told by the social system what their interactions should look like. What's more, the actual marriage ceremony is often wholly constructure to reinforce the acceptable interactions. But marriage isn't only about conscripting interactions of two individual elements, it is also an identity marker of status in the broader community. If certain elements can get married and certain elements can't, a social system has narratives around who deserves access to resources and who doesn't. Historically and currently, many LGBTQ individuals have been denied access to marriage and its accompanying privileges. The restriction of marriage in a social system is created by a narrative saying who deserves privileges and who doesn't.

Assessing the context of the family helps the therapist answer "why" questions. The context tells us why the family has the current rules of interactions; it can tell us why certain individual elements take certain roles; it can tell us whether the family has been denied resources based on their social identities and if this denial of resources is reflected in their physical environment. Social systems are also what typically create competition of autonomy within families. All family "problems" are connected to context. Systems don't have to compete for autonomy if there are sufficient physical and emotional resources. The scarcity of emotional and physical resources is often the result of social systems and the narratives that are used to allocate emotional and physical resources. The rules of interactions often get stressed and systems compete because the context is asking too much of the system or because the historical context in which the family system has adapted doesn't fit its present context.

Gathering Information

But how do you get this information? Getting the right information about the elements, purpose, interactions, and context is key to a good systemic diagnosis. There isn't one way to do this, but I want to try to make it easy until you develop your own style of gathering the important information and we'll discuss this more in Chapter 8. As you'll see in Figure 5.1, I've provided some questions that could guide you in gathering good information when interviewing an individual; in Figure 5.2, I've provided potential questions to ask when interviewing a couple; and in Figure 5.3, I've provided questions you could ask when interviewing

EPIC Questions for Individuals

Elements

When you think about the issue that brings you to therapy, who are the people in your life that are most relevant to this issue?

Regarding the issue that brings you to therapy, is there someone that it effects other than you?

When you struggle with the issue, who do you turn to? Who is helpful? Who isn't?

Is there someone or a specific relationship where the issue doesn't happen?

Purpose

When the issue does happen within one of your relationships, how does that affect your other relationships?

Do you think there are certain relationships that are more affected by this issue than others?

When the issue is affecting your relationship with _____ , how does that change your relationship with the other people in your family?

Interactions

When the issue comes up, what happens between you and _____ first? Then what happens? How do they respond? How do you respond?

Do you think _____ and _____ would describe your relationship with them the same way? Or how do you think it might be different?

Do you notice a pattern that happens repeatedly in your relationship with _____ ? How about in the relationship between _____ and _____ ? Or between all three of you?

Context

Do you think your relationship with _____ would be different if your roles were reversed? How so?

How does the community you live in shape the issue you are bringing to therapy?

How do your religious beliefs or your family's culture shape the issue that brings you to therapy?

Do you feel like your gender (or race, age, ability status, financial situation) impacts the issue that brings you to therapy?

Figure 5.1 EPIC questions for individuals

a family. Again, this isn't what you have to ask clients, but hopefully it will give you an idea of possible questions that can help you gather information. Also, these questions are just starting points, typically you are going to need to follow-up on the answers that clients provide. The initial questions you ask are typically more about the narrative that has been developed to justify the interactions after the fact. Your goal is to see beyond the narrative and into the patterns of the system.

As I said before, these aren't the questions that must be asked – they are just suggestions. You'll also notice that some of the questions that are listed in the family section could be asked to the individual; some of the

EPIC Questions for Couples

Elements

Regarding the issue that brings you both to therapy, are there other people that it affects?

Besides the two of you, who else is in your family? Who is it important for me to keep in mind when talking about this issue?

Are there people close to either of you who tend to make this issue worse or better?

Purpose

How does this issue affect your relationship with other people who are close to you and your marriage (relationship, etc.)?

If this issue results in a conflict between the two of you, who is the person you are most likely to talk about? Do they tend to help you two or does it cause more problems?

When this issue arises, do either of you pull someone in for help?

Interactions

When you are experiencing the issues between the two of you, who notices first? How do you bring it to the other person's attention?

When your partner brings it to your attention, how do you respond? What's going through your mind when it's brought to you?

When you bring up this issue to someone outside of your relationship, does this affect the relationship between that person and your partner? How so?

Context

Do you think there is a power imbalance in your relationship? Do you feel this affects that pattern?

What about the other important people in your family, do you feel that they have more power when it comes to this pattern?

How has your relationship evolved since you met? What is different about it now than when you first met?

What about the other people close to you, how have your relationships with them changed over time?

Figure 5.2 EPIC assessment questions for interviewing a couple

EPIC Questions for Families

Elements

I know we've got a good representation of your family here, is there anyone missing that you think should be here?

Who else is an important part of this family that I need to keep in mind as we talk today?

When you all think about the issue that brings everyone to therapy today, is there someone who isn't here that would have a unique perspective on what's going on?

Purpose

When you think about all of the relationships in your family, what relationships have biggest points of conflict or tension?

What two people in this room get along the best? The worst?

If there is conflict, what three people is it most likely to involve? Who would be left out?

Interactions

When _____ and _____ are getting along, what do they do? When you see that, what do you do?

When _____ and _____ aren't getting along, what do they do? When you see that, what do you do?

Do you have rules in your family that no one talks about? What are they? How do you know they are rules?

Context

Who is "in charge" in your family? Who has the most say on what happens and what doesn't?

Do certain people get treated differently in your family? Why does that happen? When does this happen?

Does your family have religious or spiritual beliefs? How do these affect how you understand the issue that brings you to therapy?

Do you think your role in the family would be different if your age (gender, financial status, etc.) was different?

Figure 5.3 EPIC assessment questions for interviewing a family

questions that are listed in the couple section could be used with a family. These questions aren't exclusive to the configuration of elements that shows up in your therapy room. Really, I just wanted to give you some examples to hopefully help you create your own process.

Sometimes you'll get good information, but with so many elements and interactions it can be hard to keep track. To help you keep track, I've created a template to document the information you gather (see Figure 5.4). You don't have to use this document, but I find it can be a helpful way to organize the information you collect. As you get more comfortable gathering information to create a systemic diagnosis, you may find this

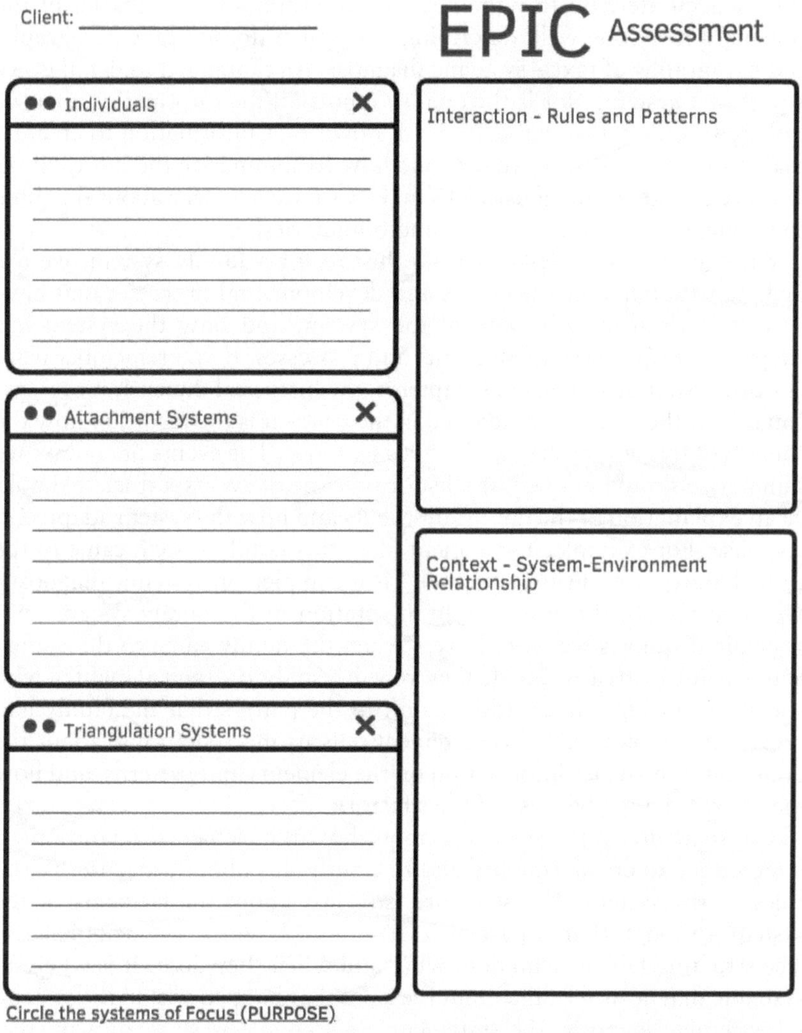

Client: _____   # EPIC Assessment

● ● Individuals   ✕

_____
_____
_____
_____
_____
_____
_____

● ● Attachment Systems   ✕

_____
_____
_____
_____
_____
_____

● ● Triangulation Systems   ✕

_____
_____
_____
_____
_____
_____

Interaction - Rules and Patterns

Context - System-Environment Relationship

Circle the systems of Focus (PURPOSE)

Figure 5.4 EPIC assessment sheet

document a bit incumbering. To me, that's a good sign. As you practice and improve your ability to gather information, it becomes second nature. Hopefully, these tools can be a way that helps you get there.

Systemic Diagnosis – The State of the System

The information we gathered through EPIC allows us to describe the state of a family system. If we gather information well, we should be able to accurately portray the history, structure, and boundaries of the system. When done well, describing the system doesn't take paragraphs and paragraphs of text – systemic diagnosis isn't intended to detail every aspect of a system. Nor is the goal to report all the information that we gathered. Rather, the goal is to distill down that information to create a usable summary. Before we describe how to summarize the information to make a systemic diagnosis, let's make sure we are clear about the three components – history, structure, and boundaries.

When it comes to describing the history of a family system, we are looking to summarize the events and developmental processes that have occurred within and outside of the system, and how the system has adapted in response to these events and processes. If you remember from our discussion of systems in Chapter 4, the historical dimension of a system is how the system has adapted in the past – it is the record of how the context of the system shaped the rules within it. The events or context we summarize should not be just a list or timeline of events; rather, it should be an explanation of the important events and how the system adapted in response. For example, a statement like "this family system came to the United States from Eritrea in 2004," is incomplete in systemic diagnosis. We want to link this event to an adaptation in the family system. In a systemic diagnosis we would say, "when the family came to the United States from Eritrea in 2004, they relied heavily on their daughter who was fluent in English, creating a shift in the patters that the family had previously employed." This statement tells us more than just about the event, but it provides information on the elements and patterns, and how they have adapted because of their history.

The structure of the system is about how the elements organize their interactions to create stability and flexibility. It's about the patterns and rules of the system. The structure isn't just about the elements of the system – though that is part of it. It's about how the elements behave. The structure tells us who does what and when they do it. It is where in systemic diagnosis we talk about the rules that happen within the system. In systemic diagnosis, the statement "this couple is stuck in a pursue-withdraw pattern" would be incomplete. Using the context provided by the history of the system, then we describe the rules of multiple elements of a system. So instead of saying "this couple is stuck in a pursue withdraw pattern" we would say,

> due to an affair that occurred two years prior, this attachment system has developed a stabilizing pattern that has the partner who cheated constantly reaching for connection, and the other partner pulls back at any bid for connection. When the partner who cheated gives up, this partner turns to their mother for a sense of belonging. After they talk to their mother, they get a sense of calm and stop pursuing the other partner. This leads the other partner to feel that something is

off, and this partner begins pursuing. When the other partner reaches for the partner who cheated, that partner mentions the conversation with the mother, and the other partner gets upset and claims the cheating partner has broken the trust again. The other partner pulls away and the cheating partner resumes pursing.

This type of statement connects history to the current structure. It expands beyond a dyad to include a triangulation system. It tells you about the rules and patterns of the system and how the elements within the system behave.

The boundary of the system is about how it interacts with the environment and the social systems in which it is embedded. If the history of the system tells us how a system has adapted, the boundary of the system tells us how it is adapting, or not, now. The boundary of the system is how the rules of the system distinguish the system from other systems – or elements within the system from other elements. The boundary of the system regulates the exchanges with the environment. In the case of a family system, this isn't only the physical environment, but also the social environment. In systemic diagnosis we wouldn't just say something like, "the family lives in an unsafe neighborhood." This statement is devoid of the context and understanding of social systems that creates "unsafe" neighborhood. What's more this statement tells us nothing of the boundary – how the family interacts with the neighborhood it's embedded in. Rather, it just tells us what the therapist thinks about the neighborhood. A systemic diagnosis statement about the boundary of a system would read something like,

> this family lives in a rapidly gentrifying community – many of their neighbors have recently moved after their rents were increased. This family used to have a strong sense of community that allowed them to feel connected and safe to those around them, but as the neighborhood has changed, so has their boundary with it. This family now is more aware of how they act in public, worried that their neighbors might see them as problematic and call the cops. They rarely connect with neighbors anymore and find themselves more isolated.

This statement talks about how the family interacts with their environment, not just about the environment. When describing a boundary of a family system, it is important to think about the interaction, and how a family regulates that interaction. Not just the environment itself. Often, our assumptions about how a family interacts with their physical and social environment can make us miss important information about the system.

Good systemic diagnoses include all three of these components – statements on the history, structure, and boundary of the system. Many times, these statements overlap with each other, but a good systemic diagnosis will detail each in a way that paints a clear picture of the state of a system.

To illustrate this, I want to provide you with another template for making systemic diagnosis. As you'll see, it's simple. It encourages you to distill the information you've put into your EPIC assessment document to make brief statements. Like I mentioned before, this doesn't need to be an exhaustive description of each rule or pattern in the system, all the developmental context, or even each element or point of competing conflict. Rather, the goal is to develop clinical judgment to determine which ones are the most relevant. Again, I've created another worksheet to help you do that (see Figure 5.5).

I'm guessing as you are reading this, systemic diagnosis may seem a bit abstract. That's okay. I'm not expecting you to wrap up this chapter and feel confident to gather good information and make an accurate systemic diagnosis. I want to help you begin to do that throughout the rest of the book. In Chapter 6, I'm also going to talk more about systems with thriving and disintegrating trajectories, to help give you language to add to your systemic diagnosis. I know we've covered a lot of ground in this chapter, so before we move forward and develop the skills to make systemic diagnosis, I want to recap the main ideas of this chapter. Hopefully this summary will help these ideas stick as we move to the next part of the book.

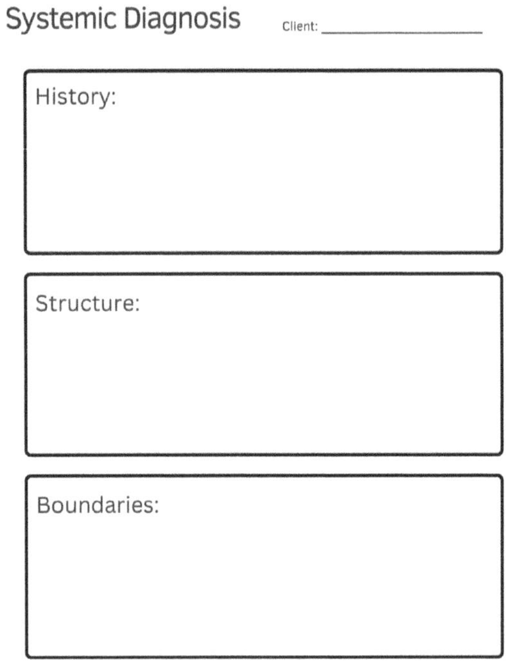

Systemic Diagnosis   Client: _____

History:

Structure:

Boundaries:

Figure 5.5 Systemic diagnosis worksheet

Recap: Main Ideas and Arguments

1. Case conceptualization as currently practiced in family therapy is often atheoretical or intervention driven. Without a theory driving the diagnosis or conceptualization, therapists are creating their own "theories." These theories are typically ad hoc explanations of what they saw. Instead of setting parameters that help therapists focus on what is important, these ad hoc explanations can be more about what the therapist thinks they can do to intervene.

2. Systemic diagnosis is theory driven. It is rooted in family systems theory. Family systems theory is an evidence-based theory, built on the assumption that the family is a biological system embedded in a social environment. It hypothesized that the family is an autonomous and adaptable system.

3. Systems on thriving trajectories are flexible and robust. When pressures from the environment are exacerbated, these systems adjust to reduce the pressure – sometimes these adjustments are permanent and sometimes they occur only for a short period of time. Systems on thriving trajectories will use structural interactions to push back against pressure from the environment. These systems slow the pace of adaptation to not lose their constitutive integrity.

4. Systems on disintegrating trajectories are rigid or chaotic. If a system is on a pathway to disintegration, it may be too flexible – reacting strongly to any pressure from the structure or environment. It may make changes quickly that quell short-term stress but create unsustainable interactions or an unsustainable boundary with the environment. A system on a disintegrating trajectory may be too rigid. Structural, developmental, or environmental pressures may necessitate adaptation, but the system refuses to or can't adapt.

5. Systemic diagnosis is a description and explanation of the history, structure, and boundaries of a family system. Systemic diagnosis uses family systems theory to gather relevant information about a system and use this information to provide an account of the state of the system. To create this account, a therapist must gather information about the elements, purpose, interactions, and context of the system. The information gathered about these factors is used by a therapist to make statements about the history, structure, and boundaries of the system.

Chapter 6

Systemic Diagnosis

From Information to Application

I've found that when I talk about systemic diagnosis, the question I get asked the most is, "So, how do I intervene with a system that I've diagnosed?" My typical response is, "I don't know." And that response is not just me being cheeky – I really don't know. There are many great intervention models out there that have shown to be effective at reducing mental health problems, marital discord, and family conflict. I think that you could probably use any one of those models with systemic diagnosis and family systems theory. But right now, most of them are grounded in theories other than family systems theory.

I think that the two most prevalent theories currently used by family therapists are attachment theory and the postmodern critique. In my previous book, I outlined what I saw as the problems with each of these theories, and how grounding your diagnosis and intervention in these theories may limit the effectiveness of your practice. I presented what I saw as the ways family systems theory was a better theory to guide diagnosis and intervention. But in that book, just as here, I didn't spell out what I saw as the effective steps of intervention. I am doing that intentionally.

You'll notice that I keep returning to the argument that family therapists blur theory, diagnosis, and intervention. I think that that argument might be lost if I presented my own model of intervention based on family systems theory and systemic diagnosis. Like I said, the most common question I get asked when I talk about systemic diagnosis is "how do I intervene?" I worry that if I presented a model of intervention, I'd continue the pattern of downplaying or blurring the distinctions between theory, diagnosis, and intervention. And that many people reading this book would forget most of everything I argued, and just look for the next cool intervention to help them with their clients.

Another reason I don't present a model of intervention is this: I don't have one. There are people out there who are much more qualified than me to create models of intervention. My training and experience have always been more focused on theory and diagnosis, not intervention.

DOI: 10.4324/9781003295907-8

I am still clinically active – I work at the University of Iowa's hospital and clinics, and I have my own private practice. I like to think that I'm a decent clinician. But for me, my "model of intervention" isn't consistent across all my clients. It depends on the system that is in front of me. In other words, I find that my interventions must be adapted based on my systemic diagnosis. No two systems will ever be the same. But if I can make a good systemic diagnosis, I can not only see the current state of the system, but I can also envision what needs to happen to move from stuck to adaptable.

Family systems theory predicts and explains interactions in a family system; systemic diagnosis uses the assumptions and hypotheses of family systems theory to describe the family system. It also predicts where the system might end up if the structure and boundaries of the system don't adapt. To me, that's where its usefulness lies. If we can accurately diagnose a family system, then we should be able to predict what would happen if no adaptations occurred. What's more, we should be able to predict what shifts in the structure and boundaries of the system are necessary for the system to thrive. Systemic diagnosis, when done well, should help us describe what an evolved system would look like at the end of therapy. It should accurately describe the current state of the system and be a roadmap as to what the system needs to do to remove points of competing autonomy. It should make good predictions about how a system can adapt without adapting so fast that it loses its autonomy.

So instead of presenting a model of intervention, l want to guide you on how to use the information you gather through your EPIC assessment to make a clear systemic diagnosis. In this chapter, I'm not going to list off criteria or symptoms; nor am I going to detail types of families. But I am going to give you ways to categorize and conceptualize the history, structure, and boundaries of systems. I am going to introduce terms that can be useful to describe the rules of the structure of a systems boundary, but that doesn't mean that the steps of the rules or patterns of the boundaries are the same across systems. Systems are all going to develop interactions and patterns based on the unique developmental context that a family experiences. But family systems theory circumscribes the possible explanations that could decrease or increase a system's autonomy.

If you remember, in Chapter 4 I talked a bit about trajectories of family systems – thriving trajectories and disintegrating trajectories. To understand how systemic diagnosis can help us create a roadmap for intervention, we'll need to revisit and expand on some of the ideas that I presented there. So, that's where we'll start. I want to be clear about something before we jump in. I've been intentional to use the term "trajectories." A trajectory implies that a system is on a path, not a specific category. Systems adapt – it's part of what they do. Adaptation is a trajectory; one adaptation is going to lead to another and another. While the adaptation paths of systems may lead to disintegration or increased autonomy, that doesn't mean that the paths are similar. The adaptive trajectory of one system that is thriving will look very different from another; the same goes for disintegrating trajectories. In other words, I don't think we can ever specify exactly what systems with thriving trajectories and systems with disintegrating trajectories do. We can only talk about the theoretical shared characteristics of each. That's what I'm going to do here.

Disintegrating Trajectories

I don't think that all families that come to therapy are on disintegrating trajectories, but many are. Many are coming to therapy as a last resort and feeling like they have exhausted all their options to try and make things better. The narrative that many systems bring when they are on a disintegrating trajectory will often be about someone else being to blame, focused narrowly on one element or subsystem as "the problem," or it will have extremely high levels of conflict. They may even have some elements that refuse to come to therapy.

Family systems theory would predict that those systems with disintegrating trajectories would demonstrate similar characteristics in their history, structure, and boundaries. Like I said before, this isn't to say that these families share the same lived experience, that all unhappy families are unhappy for the same reason, or that their patterns or rules for interactions would be similar. Rather, it means that family systems theory circumscribes what are the potential avenues for families to be at risk of or in fear of losing their autonomy.

History of Systems With Disintegrating Trajectories

A system's history records how the system has adapted to maintain its autonomy in the past. Typically, when a family system is on a disintegrating trajectory, you'll find a history of intense contextual or environmental adaptations that solved immediate crises but later resulted in new threats to autonomy. They can include things like mass tragedies, natural disasters, war, or other crises. It's not that these adaptations to the immediate crisis were bad – many times they helped the system survive the crisis. The adaptation becomes problematic when the system doesn't or can't return to its previous patterns. For example, if a family lost a home in a natural disaster, heightening the belonging processes of the interactions through intense threat-response processes may be a smart short-term adaptation. But if the interactions within this system continue to be burdened with heightened threat-response and belonging process, it's likely that they will develop a pattern that needs the family to remain in crisis for the pattern to play out. The system learns that its autonomy is only maintained if there is a constant threat that requires intense inter-actions that try to bring the elements together. Often the current state of a system on a disintegrating trajectory reflects a history of crisis that threatens a system's autonomy resulting in intense adaptations.

The history of systems with disintegrating trajectories may also be wrought with insidiously toxic environments. Many family systems are embedded in social systems that marginalize or oppress them. Because of that, they often have long histories of adapting to these environments. When family systems must navigate systems that are plagued with rac-ism, homophobia or transphobia, sexism, or other social system narra-tives that treat them as less than or insignificant, the resulting adaptations can, over time, create points of competing autonomy within a system or stress it to the point where the boundary becomes too rigid or too fluid. What's more, often those in the social environment with power will see the adaptations that these families have made to survive the toxic envi-ronments and blame them as being dysfunctional. This serves as an addi-tional toxicity in their environment creating a never-ending pressure on some families to show that they have got everything together in a social context that never allows them to have anything together. When a system comes to therapy that is on a disintegrating trajectory, toxic environ-ments can play a key, but often overlooked, role.

Systems with disintegrating trajectories may also have histories of abu-sive rules, patterns, or interactions. This can be anything from emotional manipulation, violence or threats of violence, sexual abuse, among many others. Often systems will adapt their structures and boundaries to create protection for the one perpetrating the abuse and silence those who are experiencing it. These family systems may isolate themselves from others who could intervene to stop the pattern and create rules that maintain secrets and rigid boundaries from outside systems. These rigid bounda-ries and structures often are viewed by members of the system as key to maintaining the system's autonomy, but often lead to more intense abuse or violence in ways that manifest as mental and physical health problems. Any family system with histories of abuse, neglect, or violence will be on disintegrating trajectories. While those with power in this system may view these rules and patterns as key to the systems autonomy, abuse, neglect, or violence will almost always result in disintegration.

But not all systems on disintegration trajectories have trauma, or abuse, or reside in toxic environments. Some may have just failed to adapt to the developmental or environmental changes that have occurred. They may be stuck with rules and patterns that worked at a certain point in the system's history or development but now reflect something that can sustain the system's autonomy. It may be that if they keep these patterns, the trajectory may result in abuse, trauma, or something else that results in intense stress on the system. Or it may be that there is a violation of the system's historical boundaries that occurred (e.g., an affair or a member of the family leaving a religious community) and has created chaos or upheaval in the rules of the system. While not all systems on a disintegrating trajectory have abuse, trauma, or toxic environments, all systems with disintegrating trajectories have rules or patterns of interaction that are no longer suited to the current environment or development.

Structure of Systems on Disintegrating Trajectories

The rules or patterns of a system are the systems structure. They tell the elements of the system what, when, and how to interact. If a system is on a disintegrating trajectory, then the current rules and patterns may be poorly suited to the environment, but they are also a known entity. Because the structure of the system is a structure that the system is familiar with, changing those rules and patterns can be seen as a threat to the system's autonomy – even though the opposite is occurring.

If you remember from Chapter 5, when talking about the EPIC assessment, I introduced three broad categories of rules or interactions – homeostatic, flexibility, and boundary rules. We'll cover the last rule in just a bit, but the first two types of rules – homeostatic and flexibility – are rules that pertain to the structure of the system. Systems on disintegrating trajectories still have homeostasis and flexibility rules; these rules, however, often create points of competing autonomy.

In case you forgot, homeostasis is what establishes and enhances internal functioning. Homeostatic rules use threat-response, belonging, and individual processes to generate interactions to maintain a constant internal environment. Flexibility rules are about reversible and irreversible changes to interactions. Flexibility reflects a system's ability to generate answers to conditions or changes in the environment. These rules reflect how a system adapts during a crisis or how a system changes over time. Flexibility rules specify what types of changes can happen in the threat-response, individuality, and belonging processes and what types cannot.

For family systems on disintegrating trajectories, their homeostatic rules often divide out the threat-response, belonging, and individuality processes. For example, a common homeostatic rule in an attachment system is a pursue-withdraw pattern. In that rule, one person is often responsible for keeping the two elements together – belonging processes. The other person is responsible for keeping the elements separate – individuality processes. The person responsible for keeping the elements together pursues and the one responsible for keeping the separateness or autonomy of each element withdraws. The more each element gets calcified in its role, the more anxiety or threat-response processes are infused into the cycle. This anxiety cements the rule as something that is necessary to the system's internal functioning and thereby necessary for autonomy.

Homeostatic calcification also happens in a family's triangulation systems. If an attachment system has a pursue-withdraw homeostatic pattern, this often results in triangles that are used to manage the anxiety of that pattern. The pursuer may enlist another element in another attachment system to quell the fear of the loss of autonomy. This other element may develop the role of being the intermediary between the other two elements. This might be done by being the "go between" being "the problem" or by being the "peacemaker." Often, instead of reducing the anxiety of the attachment system, the polarization continues. If the third element in the triangle is "the problem," they have to continue being "the problem" or the "peacemaker" or the "go between." The homeostatic rule of the triangle is that each element must do their part to keep the interaction going. While this often undermines the system's autonomy, the system continues because it may have worked previously.

For systems on disintegrating trajectories, the calcification of the homeostatic rules reduces a system's ability to be flexible. If we apply this idea to the family system we discussed earlier (with the pursue-withdraw rule in the attachment system and triangulations system rules of "the problem"), we can see the connectedness of the homeostasis and flexibility rules. The calcification of the pursue-withdraw rules creating a calcified "problem" rule in the triangle reduces a system's ability to respond to the environment. The flexibility rules must then polarize to one of two places – rigidity or chaos. In either location, the homeostasis rule remains the same; the difference is in who can enact the roles necessary to complete the rule. In systems with rigid flexibility rules, the elements must remain in the same roles to maintain the homeostasis rule. In systems with chaotic flexibility rules, the interactions of the homeostatic rules must remain, but the elements or systems that carry them out can change. In rigid systems, the pursuer must remain the pursuer, and the withdrawer the withdrawer. In chaotic systems, the pursuer could be the withdrawer and the withdrawer could be the pursuer – it doesn't matter which elements play the role, it just matters that it gets played.

When this polarization occurs, making reversible or irreversible changes based on fluctuations in the environment becomes nearly impossible. A system's flexibility rules are connected to its homeostatic rules. If a flexibility rule threatens the internal stability of a system, then flexibility rule become polarized. In other words, the rules of homeostasis affect the rules of flexibility. The calcification of the homeostatic rules means that there are limited options for the system to be responsive to its environment.

Calcification and polarization of a system's rules undermine its autonomy, creating points of competition between elements and systems. When the homeostasis or flexibility rules of a family system generate competition between the elements for their autonomy that is when the disintegration begins. Competition for autonomy is often described as conflict, arguments, or fights. But the competition isn't just between individual elements. Attachment elements can feel threatened by other attachment systems; triangles can be threatened by other triangles. When assessing the sources of competing autonomy, often the focus is on individuals, but the structure of systems on disintegrating trajectories often creates tension within other systems within the family system. As the elements and systems compete because of the calcification and polarization of their rules, the structural integrity of the system begins to tear, often leading to greater competition.

Boundaries of Systems on Disintegrating Trajectories

The structure of the system – it's homeostasis and flexibility rules – shape and are shaped by a systems boundary. A boundary of a system is created by the separation from the environment rules. If you remember from Chapter 5, these rules govern how a system keeps the environment outside of the system. Without these rules, the environment may overwhelm the system, resulting in the system losing its autonomy. However, the system can never be fully differentiated from its environment, so separation rules also regulate exchanges with the environment. The threat-response, individuality, and belonging processes that occur in the elements of a system help the system stay connected to the environment without being overwhelmed by it.

If a system has a calcified and polarized structure, the social or physical environment can overwhelm it. Often, systems on disintegrating trajectories experience changes in their environment as threats. Their calcified homeostasis rules have led to polarized flexibility rules, so any shift in the environment means there is no way to renegotiate the boundary between the system and the environment. Rigidity or chaos may look like renegotiation, but it isn't. Renegotiation would require making reversible and irreversible changes within the acceptable range of homeostasis. Because there is no room for flexibility, the failure to renegotiate the boundary can exacerbate the points of competing autonomy, leading to greater perceived threats to homeostasis and greater disintegration. As the environment stresses the points of competing autonomy, it begins to overwhelm the system.

However, the reverse can also occur. As I discussed before, sometimes the environment is so overwhelming that it forces calcification and polarization of the structure. Toxic environments can overwhelm a system. The system may have homeostasis and flexibility rules that help it adapt to changes in the environment or developmental context. But if those changes are too great, they can create competing autonomy between elements and thereby calcify and polarize the structure.

When either of these scenarios are occurring the rules for separation reflect the structure. Boundaries of systems on disintegrating trajectories are using separation rules that are rigidly calcified, or chaotically calcified. Whenever the environment necessitates a renegotiation, a system with a disintegrating trajectory will either refuse to adapt by keeping everything the same or refuse to adapt by giving elements new responsibilities but not changing the homeostasis rules. Often when this is the case, the system is frequently under duress as there are no meaningful exchanges with the environment. Instead, any change in the environment is seen as a threat requiring immediate action from an unadapting system, resulting in more calcification and polarization through the systems threat-response processes.

Systems on disintegrating trajectories share these common characteristics. They often have adaptation histories that have led to calcified homeostasis rules and polarized flexibility rules. These rules make any exchange with the environment feel threatening. That isn't to say that the steps or actions of the rules are the same – not every polarized and calcified attachment system will have a pursue-withdraw pattern. The interactions that create the rules can vary widely. As we'll discuss in later chapters, deciphering the steps of the rule is important. But no system is going to have the same rules. While their rules may share characteristics, that doesn't mean that the interactions are the same.

Thriving Trajectories

It would be easy to think that systems with thriving trajectories are just the opposite of systems with disintegrating trajectories. But this isn't the case. Systems on these two trajectories are not opposite, but they are different. In many instances, systems with thriving trajectories have histories marked by trauma or tragedy, hold marginalized identities, and are in toxic environments. They may even have pursue-withdraw patterns, times of chaos or rigidity, and sometimes the way they negotiate exchanges with the environment might be poor. Systems with thriving trajectories aren't perfect – they are adaptable. What makes these systems different than systems with disintegrating trajectories is how they adapt. Instead of being calcified, polarized, and overwhelmed by social, developmental, and environmental changes, thriving systems are robust and flexible.

Robustness

Robust can be a stand-in word for healthy – and I guess you could argue that this is the case in family systems theory in some respects. But when I argue that systems on thriving trajectories are robust, I'm talking about their history and structure of the homeostasis rules. We talked a bit about robustness in Chapter 4 when talking about biological systems. But I want to expand on that concept here. In *The Origin of Autonomy*, Bernd Rosslenbroich spends time defining and giving examples of robustness and its relationship to biological autonomy. He writes:

> Robustness is concerned with maintaining the possibility of a system to function rather than maintaining an actual state of a system. . . . A system is robust as long as it maintains functionality, even if it transits to a new steady state or if instability actually helps the system cope with perturbations. Such transitions between states are often observed in organisms when facing stress conditions. One such condition can be extreme dehydration, to which some organisms can react with a dormant state, becoming active again on rehydration. These examples of extreme robustness under harsh stress conditions show that organisms can attain an impressive degree of robustness by switching from one steady state to another rather than trying to maintain a given state.

Rosslenbroich relates what he describes as principles relevant for maintaining and establishing robustness. He writes:

> One strategy to protect against failure of a specific component is to provide for alternative ways to carry out the function the component performs. This can be called 'redundancy of components.' At the genetic level, this backup strategy or 'genetic buffering' (Hartman et al., 2001) might be brought about by duplicate genes with identical roles or by different genes that constitute alternative but functionally overlapping pathways. In contrast to redundant systems in engineering, however, identical genes that do not diverge in functionality or regulation would not survive in evolution. Instead, structurally different entities perform overlapping functions, which seems to be a common principle in organisms, on other levels in addition to the genetic.

There is lots of jargon and ideas to unpack here, so let's take them one at a time, starting with the definition of robustness. As I see it, robustness in family systems theory is the adaptation of homeostasis rules across time. If you remember, systems with disintegrating trajectories often have calcified homeostasis rules. But if a family system has robust homeostasis rules, it can transition to new steady states. Robust homeostasis rules also allow for the family system to use instability to adapt to environmental threats. This doesn't mean that the rules are overly malleable and change quickly. Rather, it means that a family system with a thriving trajectory will have a history of responding to crisis and being able to transition back to its previous state before the crisis. For example, if a family experiences the loss of employment by one or more of its members, if the homeostasis rules are robust, they will be able to transition to a state that is different than the previous state. They have made an intense, short-term change. But instead of making this new, intense, short-term change the new homeostasis, it is only transitory. If a family member is reemployed, the system can transition back to its previous state. It won't necessarily be the exact state – the instability it experienced will help it cope with stress in the future.

How family systems do this is embedded like the principle of maintaining robustness that Rosslenbroich describes. If you remember, I argued that in disintegrating trajectories, one element is often responsible for a single process – one element becomes the "pursuer" and one the "withdrawer." This splitting up of functions is part of calcification. But in thriving trajectories there is "redundancy of components" or the ability of any element to activate or engage the threat-response, individuality, or belonging processes. The elements of systems on thriving trajectories can overlap or have flow between individuality and togetherness. One element is never the pursuer nor is an element the withdrawer. No one element becomes the "anxious one" responsible for threat-response processes. Rather, elements can overlap and help each other carry out the steps of the rules. Instead of competition there is cooperation.

As I argued earlier, systems with thriving trajectories aren't problem free but the robustness of their homeostasis rules allows them to respond differently than families with calcified rules. And research bears this out. In my first book, I make this argument using the research of Tamara Afifi and her colleagues. They looked at how families responded to a large environmental and social change, the great recession of 2007–2009. I wrote:

> Afifi and her colleagues (2016) noted that some families 'uplifted each other, were unified in combating the recession, were present emotionally and communicatively, and blamed outside forces (e.g., government, banks, great recession). These families were more likely to bounce back following a large environmental stressor.' Other families, 'became stuck in intractable cycles of conflict where they perceived each other as a threat and communicated in ways (e.g., criticism, contempt) that preserved the self rather than the other person or the relationship.' These families were more likely to break up through divorce or conflict.

Families that were able to thrive during the recession were ones that had robust process and interactions. Those that didn't had calcified interactions that led to reactions to shifts in the environment that served only to increase the threats to their autonomy.

Flexibility

Systems with thriving trajectories are not only robust but they are also flexible. If you remember, systems on disintegrating trajectories have flexibility rules that are polarized; they are either rigid or chaotic. But systems on thriving trajectories have flexibility rules that are, pardon my redundancy, flexible. Let's return to Rosslenbroich's writings to illustrate this. When talking about flexibility, he wrote:

> Flexibility of behavior allows the [system] to find its own solution for problems and tasks or even to act independently from external necessities. . . . The essential point is that new actions can be generated and practiced. This position also takes into account that the variety of possible answers to the same environment is larger than necessary at any particular moment. . . . Increased flexibility of behavior was generated during evolution by way of the principle of uncoupling. Beginning with the generation of simple nervous systems, sensory stimuli were uncoupled from reactions, which subsequently could be increasingly modulated. Mere reflexes are still closely coupled to sensory input.

Let's unpack that a bit too. Rosslenbroich defines flexibility as a system's way of finding its own solutions. Flexibility assumes that there are a variety of ways to respond to changes in the environment or to internal pressures. The reason that some systems can be flexible is because of uncoupling. Uncoupling is the evolutionary process of making it so that species with increasing autonomy are required to immediately activate their threat-responses when a change is perceived. Reflexes would be an example of a process that hasn't uncoupled – like flinching when something flies toward your faces. Reflexes aren't bad – in some cases they can save our lives – but they don't allow for flexibility. By uncoupling responses from sensory input, systems can be flexible.

The flexibility rules of systems on disintegrating trajectories are polarized – they are either rigid or chaotic. In some senses, they are just reflexes. When a stimulus is detected, we have the same elements do the same things or we do the same thing just with different elements. But in systems with flexible flexibility rules, stimulus and response are uncoupled. In thriving trajectories, systems can use a variety of possible responses to changes. These responses are limited by the resources, history, and homeostasis rules, but they aren't reflexive. Systems with flexible flexibility rules can respond in multiple ways to events based on the parameters of the homeostasis rules and how they have adapted in the past.

Uncoupling also helps systems on thriving trajectories learn from poor adaptations. If a system responds to a change in the environment in a way that becomes problematic, the system then uses that new information to alter the response. It doesn't mean that it will totally abandon that response in the future – that response may be important for a future context. But the system can learn that this response and this time isn't useful for the system. If a system's structure is calcified and polarized, the ability to learn is greatly diminished. A system on a disintegrating trajectory may cling to a previous rule and be reflexive because that rule worked once in the past.

Regulated Exchanges

Systems with robust and flexible rules have boundaries that allow for regulated exchanges in the environment. These rules can help them navigate even the most toxic of environments. If the system is embedded in a social environment where the narrative serves to marginalize one or more of their identities, these systems can enlist their robust and flexible rules to push back against the toxicity. These systems often will enlist others with similar identities to buffer against the toxic environment and create communities that allow them to escape toxicity – if only temporarily. The community building serves as an adaptation that fosters rest from the toxicity that may require constant monitoring of the environment.

These systems' robust and flexible structures can also help deconstruct the toxic narratives that the social system prescribes to them. Because these systems can uncouple and have redundancy, the polarized or calcified narratives that are forced upon them by the social system are so foreign to their experience that they can see the narratives for what they are – a way to allocate resources and maintain power. While these narratives are an unjust burden, these systems not only challenge them for themselves but teach their communities about them. This can result in communities growing stronger, amassing more power, and using that power to shift the social narratives. Often those in power do everything that they can to re-calcify those narratives and dismantle those communities. Yet, in many cases, these systems use their structures to be resilient to injustice.

An example of this in the United States is the advancement of LGBTQ rights. The social narratives regarding queer people have consistently been that of marginalization and erasure. Throughout history, those in the queer community have shown remarkable robustness and flexibility and use this to create community spaces of safety. One such place was the Stonewall Inn. Police raided this space the community had created, and the patrons fought back. In response to this raid, thousands began protesting and the clash with police continued for six days. The protests along with the organizing and community building that occurred in the 1950s and 1960s helped form the gay liberation movement of the 1970s, resulting in the creation of organizations that are still in existence today (e.g., the Human Rights Campaign). While the social narratives surrounding queer individuals are still those of marginalization and erasure (this is especially true today of trans and nonbinary individuals), the community, flexibility, and robustness that these people shown had led to powerful changes in social narratives. In 1996, only 27% of people in the United States supported same-sex marriage. In 2021, that number had risen to 70% (McCarthy, 2022).

Like those on disintegrating trajectories, systems on thriving trajectories don't have the same interactions that create their rules – the steps or patterns of robust and flexible rules can vary widely. But all of them show flexibility and robustness. That doesn't mean that systems on thriving trajectories don't experience hardship, conflict, or toxic environments, or adapt poorly to their current context. However, because they have redundancy of components, can uncouple threat from response, and can use their boundaries to create community, they navigate changes within and without the systems which allows the system to maintain autonomy and, in some cases, increase it.

Systems Diagnosis and Disintegrating Trajectories

While not all people who come to family therapy have systems on disintegrating trajectories, I assume that the vast majority do. Assuming this allows for you to take the information gathered through the EPIC assessment and create a theory-driven, concise systemic diagnosis. The information you gather about the elements, purpose, interactions, and context can all be pulled together through family system theory's assumptions regarding systems with disintegrating trajectories. These theory-driven assumptions can help you write clear statements regarding the history, structure, and boundaries of any systems that comes to therapy.

When diagnosing the history of the system, we are looking for those places in time where the system may have begun its disintegrating trajectory. As we talked about in Chapter 5, the important things to include in your systemic diagnosis statement about the history are those things that shaped the current homeostasis and flexibility rules. The statement of the history doesn't need to include everything that has happened to the family or all of the information that you've gathered, but it does need to include what the therapist assumes are the most relevant to the rules of interaction. For example, a diagnostic statement about a systems history may say,

> In the fall of 2021, Ralph's father was killed in a car crash. Following this event, the system responded with intense belonging responses;

Ralph's husband, Tommy, began assuming responsibility for Ralph's emotions, while Ralph did the same for his mother to try and keep the system together.

This statement allows us to provide context for the statement we will make regarding the current homeostasis and flexibility rules of the system. It gives the "why" to the current structure of the system.

To summarize, good history statements should answer the following questions:

1. What events in the system's history, development, or context have had a large impact on their current structure?
2. How did these events alter the structure and boundaries of the system at that time?
3. How prevalent is the reaction to that event or context present in the current structure?

When diagnosing the structure of a system, we want to be clear about the homeostasis and flexibility rules of the system. In some cases, it may be beneficial to write a statement that outlines what the therapist sees as the step of the homeostasis rules. Other times, the therapist may want to instead provide more of an overview of the rule. If we assume the system is on a disintegrating trajectory, we are going to assume that the homeostasis rules are calcified. The intensity of this calcification can vary by system, but we should be able to assume that there is a pattern that occurs repeatedly that is creating points of competing autonomy. For example, you may describe homeostasis rule by saying something like,

> Since the death of Ralph's father, the homeostasis rule has reflected changes made during that time. Ralph will often disappear to his mother's house without telling Tommy. When he finally returns, Tommy is upset, and he and Ralph argue. The argument ends with Tommy feeling guilty and Ralph saying he is not supportive. Tommy begins to over function in the relationship, which allows Ralph to feel okay about leaving to spend more time with his mother. His mother appreciates Ralph coming but often makes comments about Tommy being unsupportive. When Ralph returns home, the pattern plays out again.

This is a homeostasis rule of the system. It started as a reaction to the death of Ralph's father but has become calcified and is now the dominate pattern that is used to provide stability – even if it is undermining the autonomy of the system.

In addition to calcified homeostasis rules, it's assumed that when a family comes to therapy, they also have polarized flexibility rules. The level of polarization can vary by system, but polarization leads to rigid or chaotic flexibility rules. Like when describing homeostasis rules you may want to sketch out the steps of the flexibility rule, or you may want to give a brief overview. Either way, I think it is important to determine which pole the family is leaning toward – rigidity or chaos. I think that when describing the flexibility rule of a system it can be helpful to clarify whether the rule is rigid or chaotic. For example, you may write something like,

> Ralph, Tommy, and Ralph's mom have rigid flexibility rules. Regardless of the stress that is occurring inside or outside the system, each plays the same role in reaction to stress. When Ralph and Tommy fight, Ralph almost always is the one to leave and connect with someone else (typically his mother); Tommy almost always stays at home and figures out how he can be a better partner to Ralph; Ralph's mom almost always takes Ralph's side and criticizes Tommy.

On the other hand, if the system has chaotic flexibility rules, the statement could reflect something like this:

> When pressure is placed on the system, Tommy, Ralph, and Ralph's mom still demonstrate the same homeostatic pattern, but each person plays a different role. While Tommy never goes to Ralph's mom, he will quite frequently text an ex. When he does this, Ralph takes on the role of over functioning, and distances himself from his mother. His mother then begins to criticize Ralph for not spending time with her; this then returns the system to its typically homeostasis rule until pressure is placed on the system again.

The flexibility rules of the system typically are built on top of the homeostasis rules. They do influence each other, but homeostasis is typically the driver of the type of polarization of flexibility rules.

Good statements about the structure of the system answer the following questions:

1. What are the steps of the homeostasis rules? Which element plays which roles or functions?
2. Are the flexibility rules rigid or chaotic? If rigid, what examples demonstrate this? If chaotic, what examples demonstrate this?
3. How do the homeostasis and flexibility rules build off each other?

When making a statement about the boundary of the system we need to be clear about the history and structure of the system. The boundary of the system is created by the rules of how the system interacts with the environments. These rules are dependent on the history – how the system has negotiated its boundaries in the past, and the structure – how those negotiations have given rise to its current patterns. The system's history and current structure are what drive the rules of negotiation. When describing the boundary, we want to build off the statements we have made about the structure and history to show how the system is currently existing in their environment. That kind of statement might look something like,

> Since the death of Ralph's father and the calcification and polarization of their structure, Ralph, Tommy, and Ralph's mom have disengaged from other. Where they used to have lots of social connection, now they often either ignore or decline invitations from friends to engage socially. What's more, the church that Ralph and Tommy used to attend has taken a turn from an inclusive environment to one that is hostile towards gay couples. This also reinforced the boundaries they were already establishing leading to more rigidity and disengagement.

This statement tells us the current rules of interaction with the environment. The regulation of exchanges with the environment as currently constituted is key to understanding the system. A systemic diagnosis is incomplete if there is no diagnosis of the boundary.

Good statements about the boundary of the system will answer the following questions:

1. How does the history and structure of the system facilitate current exchanges with the environment?
2. How is the system currently negotiating its environment? What factors are key to this negotiation?

A concise systemic diagnosis, with clear statements regarding the history, structure, and boundaries of a system doesn't mean that the diagnostic process ended. Even when we've used the EPIC framework to gather information, that doesn't mean that the systemic diagnosis is complete and can never be changed. If you recall in Chapter 1, we talked about how a diagnosis is always considered a working diagnosis until the response to treatment is assessed. In other words, the accuracy of the diagnosis is dependent on the response to treatment. The same is true for systemic diagnosis. Once we've articulated the state of the system and begin to intervene, it's going to be necessary to pause and reassess the accuracy of the working systemic diagnosis. This helps ensure that we are using the additional information that gets uncovered throughout the intervention to periodically adapt our previous systemic diagnosis.

I think it's important, however, to remember that intervention and diagnosis are two separate processes. Because we need to adapt our diagnosis periodically throughout the treatment process, it can be easy to blur the lines between diagnosis and intervention. For me, the best way to adapt a systemic diagnosis is to do this outside of the therapy room. Once we have a working systemic diagnosis and begin intervention, it can become easy to alter our diagnosis based on our intervention – and not on new information that has been revealed throughout the process. I think that it can be helpful to periodically revisit the EPIC information gathering sheet throughout the course of treatment. Reviewing that sheet and then updating it based on new information that has come to light can make the distinction between diagnosis and treatment remain clear. This allows the therapist to make a diagnosis and potentially alter treatment based on the diagnosis, not the other way around.

From Calcified and Polarized to Robust and Flexible

If a family comes to therapy on a disintegrating trajectory, how do we help them shift to a thriving trajectory? How do we change calcified rules to robust ones? How do we change polarized reactions to flexible responsiveness? To make this happen, I think we need two things: a guide and tools. Without a guide and without the necessary tool to shift the structure and boundaries of the system, we can't alter its adaptation trajectory. Good guides and good tools share one thing in common – they are based on theory. If you remember, in Chapter 3, I discussed the role of theory. When it comes to intervention, theory sets the parameters of intervention. To do this it must be able to predict pathways that can result in new adaptive trajectories and have theory-driven tools that can be used to enact this. Family systems theory and systemic diagnosis can do just that.

Family systems theory provides a guide to how to help systems shift adaptive trajectories. It gives us multiple pathways to do this. If we assume that a family system comes to therapy on a disintegrating trajectory, we have multiple ways to intervene once we have made a systemic diagnosis. Let's say that a family comes to therapy, and they are totally overwhelmed by their environment, their flexibility rules are chaotic, and their homeostasis rules are intensely calcified. Family systems theory hypothesized that there are multiple avenues to shift the trajectory. We may want to create space to the family to explore their history, to talk about the events and context that led to strong shifts in their structure and boundaries. This allows greater context for the calcified homeostasis rules, which provides the opportunity to soften these rules. As the homeostasis rules soften, this allows for greater flexibility in response to the environment, leading to the system being less overwhelmed by threats in the environment. As this system has better negotiations with its environment, this allows the homeostasis rules to be robust and in turn generates greater flexibility in the system.

Or we may begin by strengthening the boundary between the system and the environment; this may result in increased flexibility to respond to pressure, leading to more robust homeostatic rules. As the homeostasis rules become more robust, the system is better able to contextualize its history and learn how it adapted in the past. We could start with any one of these factors to create a pathway to change adaptive trajectories – it doesn't really matter. But any intervention or intervention model rooted in family systems theory uses those four factors – history, homeostasis, flexibility, and boundaries. Those are the parameters that have been set for systemic intervention. There is a myriad of ways to shift those factors but for an intervention model to be systemic it must address all four. If an intervention model addresses three of these factors, it is not systemic. It must include them all.

What's more, though I've outlined pathways that could be taken, I don't really see them happening linearly. A shift in the boundaries doesn't mean we never return to help the system renegotiate those boundaries again; same goes for contextualization of the history and decalcification and depolarization of the structure. History, homeostasis, flexibility, and boundaries are all connected. As we shift one aspect, it influences others, as we use tools to intervene in one it will likely lead us to another, and potentially back to the first, or to another. But that is why it is so important to have a clear systemic diagnosis. Systemic diagnosis allows us to think through what possible shifts need to occur and what might be places to start or focus on. It allows us to see beyond broad rules and focus on specific steps of the rules or important events. It creates intentionality to the intervention that fits the system we've diagnosed. It also allows us to have an anchor point from which we can assess changes in the system. If our diagnosis of a system is accurate, we should see a change in the adaptive trajectory of the system.

The tools we use to create these changes also need to be rooted in theory. Use of the intervention tools should result in greater contextualization of the history, decalcification, and depolarization of the structure, and healthy exchange between the system and the environment. Family systems theory can be used to create parameters for tools that should be used in systemic intervention. It predicts that certain behaviors that systems engage allow them to respond flexibly to their environment and have robustness to maintain the possibility of the system. Specifically, these interventions must help the system generate what Rosslenbroich calls "complex behaviors." He writes:

> any form of complex behavior enables organisms to answer in a
> self-determined and flexible manner to signals and conditions of

their environment. This self-determination can be enhanced in some organisms, so that the answers become more flexible in the sense that the type of reaction is less fixed, and it is possible to generate new combinations of actions and reactions. The variety of possible answers to the environment is larger than necessary at any particular moment (interactive autonomy). This correlates with the evolution of more complex and sophisticated central nervous systems in different varieties of design, which increases the scope of self-referential, intrinsic functions within the system (constitutive autonomy) as more sophisticated internal processing becomes possible.

To intervene systemically, we must use tools that allow the system to generate new combinations of actions and reactions; these tools help the system develop options that are more than sufficient to respond to threats or pressure in the environment. What's more, these tools that generate complex behaviors must also develop the system's ability to adapt its structures and the rules of its structure.

Rosslenbroich argues that these behaviors are essential to increasing autonomy. He further argues that these behaviors have evolved through an evolutionary process.

Rosslenbroich argues for humans there are eight evolved complex behaviors. These are learning, play, imitation, use of tools, insight, empathy, self-awareness, and language. I want to quickly provide Rosslenbroich's ideas regarding these behaviors and how they contribute to flexible responses to stimuli, and then I want to show how many of the current interventions taught to family therapists help systems enact these complex behaviors.

Let's start with learning. He writes, "learning introduces different degrees of plasticity of behavior as different solutions for environmental problems become possible." Learning helps us identify ways to respond that we might not have previously considered. When we learn new options for responding, we are more likely to employ them.

When discussing play he argues, "play is an expression of pronounced flexibility of behavior, uncoupled from direct needs and environmental challenges. The actions reveal highly varied sequences of movement and behavior, and the sequences can even have new combinations and time structures." He notes that play is found in most mammalian species and in some birds. Play gives a chance to practice getting good at certain responses before we are intense or in fraught situations. For example, the more you play basketball and practice certain skills, the more likely you are going to perform well during a game. The play allowed you to experience the behavior without the consequences of a game.

Imitation is like play but it allows us to create flexible behavior, by watching others. Rosslenbroich writes, "Imitation reveals a flexibility in behavioral possibilities in order to follow an external example for some new behavior." We can see how others behave and imitate and learn from their responses. Tool use is another complex behavior that produces flexibility. When we use a tool we are uncoupling from reflexes. We might play with the tool to explore its usefulness and how it can be helpful in our responses.

Learning, playing, imitation, and tool use all require insight. The flexible responses we acquire through these complex behaviors don't "stick" unless there is some form of insight. Insight may be cognitive – producing new understanding, or it may be behavioral – we don't think about it, but we use it. Insight in any form is necessary for robustness and flexibility.

Empathy and self-awareness often grow out of insight. When we have insight, we can begin to understand not only our own experience but that of others. As Rosslenbroich writes, "Detachment allows the subject to experience an observed process as related to an object beyond its own internal state or even to experience itself in some objective form." When we understand our own state and the state of others, our options for responding to stimuli are increased.

If we think about these complex behaviors, it's easy to see how many of the interventions family therapists currently use help systems engage them. For example, family therapists frequently do enactments. While the way a therapist may do an enactment varies, the goal is to help the system enact many of these complex behaviors. A therapist may teach or coach a client on what to say (learning); the client may repeat what the therapist says (imitation); the process of saying the words a therapist gave them may help the client develop empathy and self-awareness. A therapist may have the family role play. As the name implies, this is a form of play that allows the family to practice responding differently to specific situations without the intense pressures that may exist outside of the therapy room.

Critiques of Current Models

When we examine family therapy intervention models most of the things that these models recommend have the goal to help families engage in these complex behaviors. However, as currently constituted, I think most of them fall short of being systemic. Remember, for a family therapy model to be systemic, it needs to address four factors – history, homeostasis, flexibility, and boundaries. With that as evaluation criteria, let's look at some commonly practiced models. I'm not going to dive deep into these models, but I do want to argue that they are not meeting the criteria to be considered systemic.

The first is Emotionally Focused Therapy (EFT). EFT is an attachment-based therapy model created by Sue Johnson. If you check out the main website for EFT (www.iceeft.com) you'll find the following as the stated goals of the three variations of EFT – EFT of individuals, EFT for couples, and EFT for families.

The goals for EFT for individuals are:

1. *To offer corrective experiences that positively impact models of self and other and shape stable, lasting change.*
2. *To offer transformative moments where vulnerability is encountered with balance.*
3. *To enable clients to move into the accessibility/openness, responsiveness and full engagement that characterizes secure attachment with others.*
4. *To enable clients to shape a coherent sense of a competent self that can deal with existential life issues and become a fully alive human being.*

The goals for EFT for couples are:

1. *To expand and re-organize key emotional responses and, in the process, the organization of self.*
2. *To create a positive shift in partners' interactional positions and patterns.*
3. *To foster the creation of a secure bond between partners.*

And the goals for EFT for families are:

1. *Accessing and expanding awareness of unacknowledged feelings associated with the family's negative pattern.*
2. *Reframing family distress and child problems within relation blocks reinforcing this distress.*
3. *Promoting awareness and access to underlying caregiving intentions and disowned attachment related needs.*
4. *Facilitating the sharing of unmet attachment needs and effective caregiving responses.*

In my reading of these goals, you can see that the goal of EFT is focused on the structure of the system – changing the homeostasis and flexibility rules. The therapist works to promote awareness of and restructure the patterns that are occurring in attachment systems. However, you'll notice that nothing is said about the history or boundary of the system. Sue Johnson has argued repeatedly that EFT is about the "here and now"; it doesn't focus on or address the past. EFT also talks very little about the social environment that these attachment systems are embedded in. To be fair others have written to try and address that critique (e.g., Guillory, 2021). But by not explicitly assessing and looking to contextualize the history or shift how the system negotiates its boundary, I don't think EFT can be considered systemic.

Not that it's trying to be. Sue Johnson has argued that attachment theory is the best theory to predict and explain human relationships. She has argued there is evidence supporting the assumptions and hypotheses of attachment theory. And I agree with her. But as I wrote in *The Science of Family Systems Theory*, attachment theory has lots of insecurities. I think that EFT would benefit from being repositioned in family systems theory. That way it could develop tools to address the history, context, and environment in ways that it currently can't. What's more, I think by being repositioned into family systems theory, it could also break away from the narrow focus of single attachment systems and develop interventions that shift patterns and structures of triangles.

Another intervention model, Structural Family Therapy, is rooted in past versions of family systems theory; however, I'd argue that because it hasn't evolved to keep up with the new evidence that has been generated over the last 50 years, as currently practiced, it isn't systemic. I think that Structural Family Therapy, as the name implies, does a good job looking to contextualize a system's history and to shift its structure, but it doesn't do much to think about how a family system's environment shapes its current context. What's more, it provides little thought into how a family could robustly push back against the environment and shape it so it is more just.

But as with EFT, some scholars are making that critique and pushing Structural Family Therapy to look beyond the boundary of the family system. If you haven't yet, I'd highly recommend you examine the critique of Structural Family Therapy that is made by Teresa McDowell, Carmen Knudson-Martin, and J. Maria Bermudez in their book *Socioculturally Attuned Family Therapy*. Not only do they provide a path for making Structural Family Therapy fit within our current understanding of family systems theory to look beyond the borders of the family, but they also do that with all the current major family therapy intervention models.

This type of work that McDowell, Knudson-Martin, and Bermudez are doing is essential to the continued development of family therapy intervention models. They are taking interventions models and critiquing them based on the new evidence that has come to light. Like them, I don't think that we need to abandon the models that have been developed but I do think we need to help them evolve based on family systems theory. I think that using family systems theory to evaluate these models based on how they addressing the history, structure, and boundaries of a system is key to keeping our interventions relevant and effective.

I also think that therapists should examine their own practice similarly. When working with your clients are you examining the history of how they adapted in the past? Do you know how these adaptations are affecting their current structure? Are you exploring their homeostasis rules? Their flexibility rules? Are you assessing the negotiations that your clients are having with their environment? Or how these negotiations are shaping the structure? To intervene systemically, you're going to need to diagnose systemically. That is why the EPIC assessment and systemic diagnostic statements are so important. They set a therapist up to intervene systemically. Intervening systemically is something I think has been disappearing from our field.

We've covered a lot of ground in this chapter as well, so next is the summary of the main ideas and arguments. Up until this point, the arguments I've made have been in support of family systems theory, systemic diagnosis, and systemic intervention. But in the next chapter, we are going to talk about the limitations. I'd recommend that before going to the next chapter, you look back over the summaries of each of the previous chapters. This will help you to weigh the evidence for and against systemic diagnosis.

Recap: Main Ideas and Arguments

1. **Systems on disintegrating trajectories often have histories, structures, and boundaries that have led to calcification and polarization.** In many cases, this results in these systems responding to any changes, pressures, or threats in the environment with intensity. This calcification, polarization, and intensity serves to create more points of competing autonomy between the elements of the system resulting in more calcification, polarization, and intensity. If this trajectory isn't changed, these systems may break apart – resulting in a loss of autonomy of what once was the entire system.

2. **Systems on thriving trajectories are robust and flexible.** These systems have redundancy of components, uncouple threat from response, and use their exchanges with the environment to build community. They are on trajectories that serve to maintain and increase their autonomy.

3. **Systemic diagnosis is key to systemic intervention.** If we don't diagnose the history, structure, and boundary of a system, it's likely that our interventions will neglect one of these components. If an intervention model does not include tools to address each aspect of the system, it shouldn't be considered a systemic intervention.

4. **The most practiced family therapy models are not systemic.** While most models address some of the components of the system, many neglect the history or the environment of the system. Many scholars have begun to address this, but much work is still needed.

Chapter 7

Potential and Pitfalls of Systemic Diagnosis

At this point, I hope that I've convinced you that family systems theory and systemic diagnosis are the future of family therapy practice. I hope that the arguments I've made regarding viewing theory, diagnosis, and intervention as separate have been clear, and you agree that lumping them together has done family therapy a disservice. I hope that I convinced you to study family systems theory and to try out systemic diagnosis in your own practice. But I'm guessing that there may be many of you who are still skeptical. Whether you are convinced or not, this is the part of the book where I point out the flaws of my reasoning and the current problems of systemic diagnosis. I do this to show you where family systems theory and systemic diagnosis fall short, but also to talk about ways these limitations could be overcome in the future.

However, if it ends up that family systems theory and systemic diagnosis can't overcome these limitations, then we'd need to abandon it. If that's how it ends up playing out, I'd be happy. Sure, I'd feel sad that what I thought would work and was important ended up not being so; however, if family systems theory and systemic diagnosis don't pan out, that will mean that researchers and practitioners have engaged with my work, thought critically about it, and created something better. To me, that would be a success. I've dedicated my career to the betterment of family therapy because I think it is an important avenue to make lives better. And if this work is just a step on the path to making that happen, then I'll take that as a win.

Regardless of what becomes of family systems theory and systemic diagnosis, let's map out what I see as the biggest limitations with systemic diagnosis. I'm not going to spend time detailing what I see as the limitations of family systems theory – I've done that already in my previous book. I'm just going to talk through the state of systemic diagnosis, and the road to making it have the empirical and clinical usefulness that I hope it has.

DOI: 10.4324/9781003295907-9

Lack of Empirical Evidence

The biggest problem with systemic diagnosis is the lack of empirical evidence. If you'll remember when I talked about the DSM and relational diagnosis, part of my argument for why they were problematic was because research assessing these models showed kappa values that were deemed unacceptable. If you remember kappa values tell us the likelihood that if two people were using diagnostic criteria from either the DSM or from a relational diagnosis, they will arrive at the same diagnosis. Kappa values for the DSM-5 diagnosis and for parent-child interaction problem kappa was below 0.6 – something that many have argued is unacceptable. To make a strong argument that systemic diagnosis is better than these other diagnostic frameworks, I'd need empirical evidence. As currently presented, I don't have any evidence that this process is reliable or valid. I can't compare the kappa values of systemic diagnosis to those of the DSM or relational diagnosis because I don't have them.

For many of you reading this, that may be a fatal flaw. And I get that. Why would you want to use any diagnostic method that hasn't been rigorously evaluated? Many family therapy training programs focus exclusively on evidence-based interventions. Family therapy has a long history of following gurus with great ideas with little evidence to support their claims. In some ways, in writing this book I'm doing the exact same thing. I'm setting myself up as a guru presenting a method without empirical evidence.

While I may not have evidence for the reliability and validity of systemic diagnosis, I think we have overwhelming evidence for family systems theory as presented here. That is what my whole first book – *The Science of Family Systems Theory* – was about. What's more, I think that the evidence suggests that family systems theory can better predict or explain human relationships than attachment theory or the postmodern critique. That's not to say the family systems theory is without its limitations. But I think, until a better theory comes along, it is the best we've got. While this may not be direct evidence for systemic diagnosis, it suggests that systemic diagnosis has a strong empirically supported theory from which it is derived.

Systemic diagnosis needs empirical evidence showing its reliability and validity, and I think that this can be done in a few ways. One way is to replicate the type of research that I summarized regarding the DSM and relationship diagnosis – the one presenting kappa values – for systemic diagnosis. I think that it would be important for multiple therapists to conduct assessments and make systemic diagnosis for the same families. Then, comparisons need to be made to see if these therapists arrive at similar statements regarding the history, structure, and boundaries of the system. The difficult thing about this type of research is that unlike DSM diagnosis or relational diagnosis, systemic diagnosis does not have predefined categories. The goal of systemic diagnosis isn't to say this family is a "depressed" system or an "anxious" system. But that means that each systemic diagnosis is unique to the system. So, while I think that this type of assessment of systemic diagnosis will be necessary, getting an empirical base of support will take multiple studies across multiple years.

Another way to create empirical support for systemic diagnosis is to evaluate how systemic diagnosis is related to therapeutic outcomes. One of the arguments I've made is that using family systems theory to make systemic diagnosis should result in better intervention. Better intervention would be determined by better therapeutic outcomes. I think that this type of evidence could be created by comparing outcomes of family systems in which a therapist made a systemic diagnosis to when no systemic diagnosis was made. What's more, it would be necessary to compare models of case conceptualization and systemic diagnosis in a similar way. If my arguments are correct, families in therapy in which a therapist made a systemic diagnosis should have better outcomes than families in therapy where the therapist used case conceptualization to plan treatment.

Until these types of empirical evidence exist, it will be difficult to advocate for widespread use of systemic diagnosis. But I do think that these and other evaluations of systemic diagnosis could demonstrate its effectiveness and importance. If that ends up being the case, then I think it would be necessary and important for family therapists to adopt systemic diagnosis as standard of practice.

Is This the Way Forward?

Another big issue I see with systemic diagnosis is how divergent it is from mainstream mental health diagnostic practice. There are thousands of researchers and practitioners out there who are pursuing diagnostic models focused on alleviating individual symptoms. There are some advocating for the continued use of the DSM diagnostic categories and there are others who are trying to find new and better models (e.g., NIMH RDoCs). As I argued in the first chapter of this book, these diagnostic models, rooted in the biomedical model, try to account for other "factors" like relationships and social and physical environments. They see these factors as important contributors to mental illness, but not the dominant one. The dominant factor is the individual – their genes, their nervous systems, and their personality.

Biopsychosocial models, like systemic diagnosis, wouldn't discount the fact that the individual system is important, but it doesn't assume that it is the dominant factor. What's more, systemic diagnosis posits that systems can be understood in isolation. To diagnose you must assess multiple systems and multiple elements. This argument is in opposition to models that aren't currently being pursued. But this argument isn't new. If you remember in Chapter 1, I quoted George Engel. Writing in 1977, he argued for the development of approaches like systemic diagnosis. It's nearly been half a century since he introduced this argument, but mainstream medical and mental health practice still is biomedically focused. I know that there are many who have taken his argument seriously and have pushed for biopsychosocial diagnosis and treatment.

This push hasn't really made the splash that I bet Engel and others would have hoped. Most of the money and brain power looking at mental health is coming at it from a biomedical framework. It may be that this is because the medical and mental health establishment is in a calcified homeostasis. It may be that the medical and mental health establishment is so invested in an individualized, biomedical approach that regardless of whatever new ideas come along, it is going to refuse to adapt.

Or it may be that the impact that focusing on individualized, biomedical diagnosis and treatment is better than a systemic or biopsychosocial approach. When you compare family or couple therapy interventions to individual therapy the outcomes aren't much different. In a recent review I did with Andrea Wittenborn et al. (2022) we looked at the effectiveness of couple and family interventions for depressive and bipolar disorders. While we found that generally they are effective, they weren't better than individual interventions – this is something that seems to be consistent throughout scientific literature. If these approaches are not resulting in better outcomes, then why keep doing them?

Couple and family interventions can also be cumbersome. It can be hard enough to get one person to go to therapy; it can be even harder to get a couple or an entire family to go to therapy. If these interventions aren't better than individualized or biomedical interventions, maybe couple and family therapy isn't getting its bang for its buck. In a medical and mental health system that is for profit, value for money is key. If it takes more effort to get the same outcome, is that extra effort worth it?

I'd push back against this argument in two ways. First, if you look at the review that my colleagues and I did, you'll see that the interventions that we reviewed aren't systemic – especially if you use the criteria we talked about in Chapter 6. Most just utilized a partner or family member to aid in the intervention. The two types of interventions that were closest to being systemic, emotionally focused couples therapy (EFT) and attachment-based family therapy (ABFT) are both based in attachment theory – a theory I've argued to be insufficient. In other words, I think that the reason that you don't see a difference between couple and family therapy interventions and individual interventions for things like depression is because they aren't systemic. I would argue that if we grounded our diagnostic models and interventions in family systems theory, we would see superior outcomes for things like depressive and bipolar disorders. But until we do that research, it's just speculation.

Second, the idea that couple and family therapy interventions are less efficient or more cumbersome so that they cost more money, doesn't really hold up. In the 2017 article, "The Case for Insurance Reimbursement of Couple Therapy," Robb Clawson, Stephanie Davis, Richard Miller, and Tabitha Webster point out the holes in this reasoning. They write:

> We assume that one of the reasons insurance companies do not include couple therapy as a reimbursable treatment for marital distress is because of concerns regarding increased costs. A line of research known as medical offset research examines the total cost effectiveness of certain treatments, including subsequent health care usage after receiving treatment. The medical offset research for couples who receive couple therapy shows that they experience a decrease in their utilization of future health care, reducing overall health care costs (Law & Crane, 2000). . . . The mounting evidence of a medical offset effect for couple therapy begs the question: Financially, is it in the best interest of health insurers to pay for couple therapy? Caldwell et al. (2007) provided a well-researched, conservative estimate of cost savings to health insurers who provide couple therapy for those exceeding a clinical threshold of marital distress. They found that providing marital screenings for all couples and subsequent couple therapy for those who are distressed would result in a $1.48 return over 12 months for every $1 spent by insurers. Furthermore, an overall medical offset effect (i.e., returns exceeding costs) would occur if at least 25% of the identified distressed couples began couple therapy as recommended.

In other words, if you target and treat the marital/romantic partner attachment system, over time, these couples will utilize less health care, costing insurers less money. If you think about it, family systems theory can provide a simple explanation of this. If you can help systems create flexible and robust interactions that allow them to adapt well to their environment, then there is going to be less stress on the system across time. Sure, there will be times when there is friction, but overall the system will be able to navigate developmental and environmental changes. With less burdened threat-response, belonging, and individuality process, these systems will not only have less stress, but will also have more ability to engage in behaviors and practices that are health promoting. If you set the system on to a thriving trajectory, the elements will be healthier.

That is something we do have loads of evidence for – people with healthy relationship systems live better, healthier lives. Julianne Holt-Lunstad made this case in her summary of the research of social relationships and health in 2018. After summarizing the research that details how our close relationships affect our lives, she advocates the use of a systems approach to improve health and well-being:

> A systems approach can potentially provide a substantially broader impact on public health than individual-based interventions . . . most individual-based interventions only target those deemed at high risk, i.e., those at the extreme end of the risk continuum. This approach adopts the 'theory of bad apples' rather than the 'theory of continuous improvement. . . .' The 'bad apples' approach seeks out precise tools to identify statistical outliers. Those at the extreme end are identified and labeled as deficient and in need of fixing to eliminate the problem. Although we should not ignore those on the extreme end of the risk continuum, exclusively focusing on this group has important limitations . . . it assumes that there is a dichotomous threshold effect of risk, meaning that below a certain threshold one is at risk, and above it one is not. However, the cumulative data do not support this (Holt-Lunstad et al., 2010). Rather, it is imperative that we recognize that there is a continuous dose-response risk trajectory (Yang et al., 2016) and that we do not focus attention and efforts entirely on one extreme end . . . focusing efforts on the extreme end of the risk continuum ignores a significant portion of the population. Instead, interventions aimed at the community and society levels that reach the entire risk spectrum may result in population-level shifts – thereby effecting a greater degree of change in risk.

Though most of our current brain power and money are funneled toward biomedical approaches and individualized treatment, this might not be the best course of action. More and more researchers are looking at the data and concluding that the biomedical model needs to be replaced by biopsychosocial models. We can't look only at individuals if we want to improve health outcomes; we must examine systems.

When it comes to psychotherapy, I do think that family systems theory, systemic diagnosis, and systemic intervention are the way forward. That doesn't mean that they will be the end point, but right now as I and many others look at our current mental and physical health care, we see the glaring need for improvement. To really reach the best outcomes, we need not just family systems theory, but other systems-based theories that can explain other important social systems. We need not just systemic diagnosis as presented here; we need other systemic diagnosis models that can account for the unique contexts of those other systems. We need many systemic intervention models that can be adapted to multiple settings, developmental contexts, and social systems. We need to think in adaptive trajectories, not just in "good or bad." That is how we can help create the environments, structures, and boundaries humans need to thrive.

Recap: Main Ideas and Arguments

1. **Systemic diagnosis has not been rigorously evaluated by researchers.** Though systemic diagnosis is rooted in an evidence-based theory – family systems theory – no current evaluations of the process have been made. This research is imperative before widespread use of this model is adopted.
2. **The individualized "bad apples" approach to mental and physical health care is insufficient.** More and more, researchers are examining the data and advocating for the use of biopsychosocial and systemic models to diagnose and intervene.
3. **Family systems theory and systemic diagnosis are important steps for psychotherapists to adopt systemic approaches.** We will need other systems theories and models, but as currently constituted, family systems theory, systemic diagnosis, and systemic interventions provide the best path for helping people thrive.

Part III

Systemic Diagnosis
The Fundamentals

Have you ever watched a professional athlete compete in a sport, then thought to yourself, "that doesn't look so hard." I know I have. When I turned 40, I decided to try my hand at boxing. I signed up to take some classes at a local gym. I'm not really a boxing fan, but I've seen enough clips on ESPN to figure that it would be easy enough and a good way to shake up my workout routine.

I still remember the first time I walked into the boxing gym; I was nervous but figured I could blend in. I thought I was in decent shape – I've run and done group fitness most of my life – so I figured that if nothing else I could at least fake like I knew what I was doing. But after about five minutes hitting the heavy bag, I was gassed.

Luckily for me, a trainer came over and started talking with me. She pointed out, correctly, that the reason why I was so exhausted was because I wasn't generating any power through my legs. If I really wanted to learn how to box, I needed to first learn to use my feet and legs – not my arms. I needed to start with the fundamentals and build from there.

I'm guessing at this point, your ideas of systemic diagnosis might be a bit like my understanding of boxing. You get the gist of it, but you still need the fundamentals. That's what I'm going to try and provide for you in Part III of this book.

To make a diagnosis of a system, we need to gather information about the elements, purpose, interactions, and context. The fundamental way we gather this information is through asking questions, following up on answers, and using a systems resistance to make implicit patterns explicit. That's what Chapter 8 is about. In Chapter 8, I'm going to ask you to reflect on what we've talked about so far and begin to think through questions you might ask a client who comes to therapy. I'll use the questions that I provided in Chapter 5 as a jumping off point, but I want you to be able to create questions that reflect your style as a therapist. Good questions are key to gathering good information. Hopefully if you ask good questions, you'll get good answers. However, the problem with answers is that often they reflect narratives that can deflect or hide the

DOI: 10.4324/9781003295907-10

actual interactions and context of a system. I'll walk you through ways to clarify answers and look for patterns that are present even if they are obscured by the narrative clients present. Sometimes this is easier than others, and it can be especially difficult when a system is resistant to gathering information. In Chapter 8, I'm also going to use family systems theory to help create ways to navigate and use resistances in therapy to get the information necessary to make accurate diagnoses.

In Chapters 9, 10, and 11 I'm going to provide you with examples and give you opportunities to think about how to gather information and make a systemic diagnosis. In Chapter 9, I'm going to describe a hypothetical conversation between me and a supervisee. I'm doing this to hopefully illustrate the elements, purpose, interactions, and context of a system and how that information is used to create a systemic diagnosis. In Chapter 10, I'm going to sit back and let you try your hand. I'll present a made-up therapy session between me and a new couple. Throughout this conversation I'm going to have you respond to some questions about what information is being gathered and how you can use this information to make a systemic diagnosis. In Chapter 11, I'm going to let you jump in. I'm going to just give you snippets of conversations and I want you to take it from there. I want you to map out what questions you would ask; I want you to role play or create dialogue; and I want you to have a sense of how you might do this in your therapy room.

I'm not expecting you to finish Part III of this book and feel like an expert in systemic diagnosis. But I am hoping that by reading it, you at least start to get your feet under you.

Chapter 8

Questions and Answers

I've been asked to be an expert witness in a few legal cases. The first time I did it, I was super nervous. I thought that lawyers had some magical skill of asking questions that would make me look like an idiot – if you can't tell, I've watched way too many dramatized courtroom TV shows. But that wasn't my experience. While some of the questions I was asked were intended to trip me up, most were "yes or no" questions. To the undying frustration of the opposing lawyer, I routinely answered her "yes or no" questions with "it depends."

Lawyers don't have any superpowers when it comes to asking questions. Though, I've found that most lawyers – especially trial lawyers – have thought a lot about *how* they ask questions. This is something that I think is desperately missing from how we train therapists. Most of the training I've ever received has focused mainly on questions to ensure to get the information to make a DSM diagnosis. I've also been in the audience of trainings where presenters have made lists of question therapists *shouldn't* ask. I've heard some folks argue that therapists should never ask "why" questions and should only ask "how" questions. Michael White and David Epston thought a lot about questions in their development of Narrative Therapy (if you've read my previous book, you'll see my argument as to why their approach was flawed). But overall, we don't spend nearly enough time thinking about the questions we use to gather information.

Questions

In the first part of this chapter, I'm going to talk through important things a therapist must consider about how they ask questions. I'm not going to spend time debating about whether certain types of questions should be asked or how to structure the perfect question. Rather, I'm going to argue for factors that I think should drive a therapist's interviewing process – the fundamentals of gathering information. To me this includes three things: using theory, slowing down, and reflecting. Then, I'm going to ask you to do some work. After I've laid out what I see as the important

DOI: 10.4324/9781003295907-11

things to consider when conducting an interview with a family system, I'm going to ask you to think through how you may want to use theory, slowing down and reflecting with your clients. I'm also going to have you create theory-driven questions that help you gather information in ways that feel comfortable and fit your style as a therapist. Some of these questions may be like the ones I presented in Chapter 5, but I want you to put your own spin on them. You can revisit some of the questions that I introduced in Chapter 5 and use those as a jumping off point. But I really hope you find your own voice and style when it comes to asking questions to gather information.

Using Theory

By now, it probably doesn't surprise you that I'd argue that to conduct good interviews or ask good questions you need good theory. However, in my experience, most therapists are thinking about intervention when they ask questions, not theory. When I see presenters talk about how to phrase questions, or types of questions that should never be asked, I tend to shake my head. For me, no matter how poorly phrased, there is only one type of "bad" question in therapy – a question that is not theory driven. If you want to gather good information from clients, you must have good theory, and you need to know this theory well. A bad theory will always result in bad questions, and lack of knowledge of good theory will also result in bad questions. Having no theory will just lead to a shotgun approach – asking lots of questions that are totally disconnected to hopefully get something useful. To avoid bad questions, I think there are two important habits that therapists must develop.

The first – stay informed. I started my therapist training in 2007. The knowledge we have about families and systems has changed dramatically since that time. If I stopped reading about theory, stopped staying on top of the research, I'd probably be asking questions that are based on outdated theory. In my opinion, those would be bad questions. It can be hard for a therapist to stay informed. Working as a therapist requires being present with clients, holding space for their pain, not to mention writing case notes, dealing with insurance, and all the other tasks that are needed. This is on top of all the responsibilities a therapist might have outside of their work. It can be hard to stay up to date with the current research and thinking about theory, but I think if we want to do our jobs well, we need to carve out time to do this. However, you do it – listening to podcasts, reading journal articles, or going to conferences – doesn't really matter. But creating a habit of critically examining the best available knowledge is key to asking theory-driven questions.

The second – be consistent. If you are hopping between many theories to guide your questions, it's likely that you aren't asking good questions. Becoming an expert in one theory takes lots of time and investment; becoming an expert in many theories can be extremely difficult. I think that all therapists should ground their work in a single theory and then dedicate their time to learning and growing their knowledge base about that theory. It doesn't have to be family systems theory, but if therapists are trying to know multiple theories in depth, the amount of investment it takes to stay informed could be nearly impossible in full-time practice. If you find yourself being able to jump from theory to theory, be honest with yourself – do you really know these theories enough to have them inform the questions you ask? Are you conflating theory and intervention? I think that becoming an expert on a single theory is a life-long quest – one that is key to good therapy. If you haven't chosen a theory to drive your practice, I recommend doing that sooner than later. And hopefully, since you're reading this book, I can persuade you that family systems theory is the one to choose.

Slowing Down

One of my first supervisors when I was in my master's program was Dr. Joseph Wetchler. To me, Joe was an expert supervisor. He had a deep knowledge of family systems theory and used creative ways to teach us theory. One of the first times I presented a family I was working with to Joe, I talked and talked and talked. When I finally took a breath, Joe started whistling. I looked at him funny and he asked if I recognized the song. I told him I did. So, he started singing it: Slow down, you move too fast/You've got to make the morning last/Just kicking down the cobble stones/Looking for fun and feeling groovy. If you're not familiar with this song, it's the "59th Street Bridge Song" by Simon and Garfunkel. When Joe finished singing, he didn't say anything for a bit, and then asked something to the effect of, "Do you get it?"

I did get it. I was going too fast, and I wasn't getting any useful information. I was asking a question about a topic and then jumping into the next topic the family brought up without ever digging deeper. I wasn't talking fast; I was changing topics fast – which allowed the system to hide behind its narrative. Joe wanted me to slow down and dig deeper. He wanted to help me find the patterns and rules of the system. You can only do this by going slow.

If you find that you're making systemic diagnoses after interviewing a family for ten minutes, you're going too fast. You need to slow down. When I say slow down, it's not about talking slower, or taking longer pauses between questions – it's about using questions to drill down to get the important information. Systems will readily tell you about the narratives that justify their rules and interactions, but these narratives aren't always accurate. Often narratives are used to hide or blur the rules or interactions. If you are going slow with your questions, you are going to link questions together to get past the surface level narrative of a system and start gathering information about the elements, purpose, rules, and context of a system. If you can link together questions that are theory driven, one after the other, you aren't going to be jumping from topic to topic. Rather, you are going to be focused on certain elements and purpose and exploring the context for the rules of interaction.

In the preceding section, I told you that therapists need to be informed and be consistent when it comes to theory. The same goes for pacing when asking questions. You need to become an expert on the system that is in front of you. To do that, you need to use your knowledge of theory to ask the questions that help you get the information to know the system better than it may know itself. You need to consistently stay on topic until you get the information that helps you make an accurate systemic diagnosis. If you find yourself jumping from topic to topic, you need to slow down and focus on following up. Linking questions together can help you drill down to find the interactions that are often absconded by the narrative.

What's more, if you go slow, sometimes the question you ask will manifest the points of competing autonomy and patterns and rules of the systems. If you are jumping all over the place without theory, you won't see this. But if you are asking theory-driven questions and going slow, the rules and patterns of the system will show themselves. That's when you can really start getting relevant information. When you witness an interaction and then can ask something like: "This thing that happened between the three of you just now, is this something that occurs frequently?" Or something like, "Did you both just see what happened when I asked that question? Did you notice how you both reacted to each other?" When you get to a place with a system where you can ask these types of questions, you are on the right track. It typically means that you've used theory and gone slow enough to ask the questions that provoke the system to show you its rules and patterns.

Reflecting

A theory-driven, slowed-down questioning process allows you to gather good information about the elements, purpose, interaction, and context of the system. But you need one more step – reflecting to the system the information you've gathered. This is crucial. Getting good information isn't easy, and sometimes when we think we've got a handle on the system, we may be leaving out other relevant information. If therapists take time to reflect to the system the information they have gathered, they will be able to assess the accuracy of their assessment and be able to set the stage for effective intervention.

Reflecting to the system the information you've gathered is a simple process. For me, it contains three steps. First, you start with their narrative or problem that brought them to therapy. Second, you state part of your systemic diagnosis – something about the history, structure, or boundary of the system. And third, you ask them to verify that what you are saying is accurate. It can be something like this:

> So your communication issues (what brought them to therapy) are really rooting in this unique time of your relationship – transition from raising kids to being empty nesters (something about the context) that has led to you both wanting more connection but trying to get it in ways that pushes the other person away (something about the pattern). Does that seem right to you both (verifying the accuracy of the information)?

If you've gotten a pretty good grasp on the elements, purpose, interactions, and context of the system, many times clients will say something like, "Yes, that's right, and I've never thought about it that way before."

Reflecting to clients may also shed light on information that you may have otherwise missed. If you state the problem that brought them to therapy, say something about the history, structure, or boundary of the system, and then ask clients if you got it right and they say "no," you are then in a prime position to get more information. If clients say "no" then you can ask them to tell you what you've missed. Or you could ask them to tell you how they see it differently. What's more, this allows you to slow down and drill down on specific interactions, purpose, or context of the system. It allows you to use your theory to ask better questions to get the right information.

In my work with clients, these three steps have helped me gather the information I've needed to diagnose a system. I've found that if I'm intentional about using theory, if I'm going slow, and if I am consistently reflecting to the system the information I've gathered, I can create an accurate description of the state of the system. On the other hand, I've found that when I'm not focused on theory, I tend to jump from topic to topic and never take the time to reflect to the clients the information I've gathered. This has often led me to feel really stuck when I try to intervene with clients. When I have a poor diagnosis of the system, my intervention tends to be equally poor.

Your Interviewing Style

Have you ever tried to return an item you bought online or changed your travel plans? If you have, most likely you interacted with a chatbot. These AI generated bots ask questions based on the algorithm that their coders have created. If you are reading this ten years in the future, these chatbots may be experts at asking questions, but currently they aren't very good at it. This past holiday season, we had issues with our travel plans and trying to chat with a chatbot was very frustrating. The questions that they could ask were very limited and often didn't get at what I really needed. After 15 minutes trying to get the chatbot to ask me a question that would help me get the information I needed to deal with our travel issue, I gave up and waited on the phone for a really long time.

I bring this up because I don't want you to be a therapybot. The way things are currently evolving, therapists might be replaced by bots in the future. Given the current state of AI, I'm not too concerned. As you'll see in Chapter 11, I think that using AI has great potential to help therapists practice and generate examples to see patterns. But until AI can develop the theory-driven creativity to intervene effectively with families, I'm not too worried. I do think that when therapists start out implementing a new skill into their practice, it can be a bit robotic. That's why I think it's important that therapists bring their own style and personality to asking questions. I don't want you to take the questions I listed in Chapter 5 and only use those as your options. Those questions were just suggestions. Rather, I want you to be intentional about the questions that will guide you in diagnosing the systems that you see in therapy.

To help you do this, I've created some workbook pages for you. You may be a person who doesn't like to write in books you've purchased, or, if you're like me, find it difficult to hold down a book and try to write. Don't worry, you can download PDF versions of these pages from my website (jacobpriest.com). You may also be the type of person who finds it awkward to write down responses to questions in the workbook – I'm the same. I'd rather think and talk about them with people whose ideas I respect and who will give me direct feedback. So, you can use the pages that follow in the way that best suits you and how you learn. But I do hope you will take the time to go through these pages before moving forward. To make systemic diagnoses takes work on your end. And while these pages are just the start of that work, I think it's an important place to start.

1. If you were to describe family systems theory to someone who had never heard about it, how would you describe it to them in a paragraph or less?

2. How would you recognize if you were going "too fast" when trying to gather information to create a systemic diagnosis? What could you do to help yourself slow down?

3. If family systems theory guides your questions in therapy, what are examples of questions you could ask that would get you good information about the **elements** of the system?

4. If family systems theory guides your questions in therapy, what are examples of questions you could ask that would get you good information about the **purpose** of the system?

5. If family systems theory guides your questions in therapy, what are examples of questions you could ask that would get you good information about the **interactions** of the system?

6. If family systems theory guides your questions in therapy, what are examples of questions you could ask that would get you good information about the **context** of the system?

7. If family systems theory guides your questions in therapy, what are examples of how you could reflect back information you've gathered about the **history** of the system?

8. If family systems theory guides your questions in therapy, what are examples of how you could reflect back information you've gathered about the **structure** of the system?

9. If family systems theory guides your questions in therapy, what are examples of how you could reflect back information you've gathered about the **boundary** of the system?

Answers

I hope you feel a little bit more confident about questions you could ask to gather the information you need; unfortunately, even the best questions won't always result in getting you the best information. Systems are stubborn – they love the processes that generate and maintain their autonomy. Often, they are going to answer questions in ways that push back against any changes. Sometimes that therapist is viewed as an agent that the system must adapt to, and this means that instead of being flexible the system may go for a robust, inflexible response. If the system can best the therapist, the system stays the same.

If you haven't found yourself in a situation like this, you will. You may have an element of the system that refuses to show up to therapy; you may have worked with a teenager who refuses to look at you or answer any of your questions; or you may have had a mandated client who told you that the whole process of therapy was useless. Getting responses like this, especially when you've put in the work to ask good questions, can be frustrating. You may feel like you are running into a brick wall over and over again. In my experience, when clients respond to therapists' questions with these types of answers, therapists tend to move on from diagnosis and just focus on intervention. In some cases, that may work out for the therapist. But I think that sets up a bad pattern in your therapeutic practice – one that misses diagnosis all together. You may get lucky and have an intervention that works without a proper systemic diagnosis; however, that will most likely be the exception not the rule.

When systems give rigid, inflexible responses, therapists often refer to this as "resistance." You may have heard a supervisor say something to the effect of "resistance doesn't reside in the client; resistance always resides in the therapist." That sentiment suggests that when we get stuck in therapy, it's because the therapist needs to do something different. I think that this type of thinking is problematic. Systems are supposed to resist change. Sure, they need to adapt, but this adaptation can't happen too fast (or too slowly). For a system to maintain its autonomy, it must resist. That is the whole purpose of the boundary of the system. This boundary regulates the rate of change and exchanges with the environment. In the therapeutic environment, we should expect family systems to resist by regulating the exchanges and the rate of change.

But this also means that resistance exists in all systems – even the therapist's systems. Just as clients can regulate exchanges with their environment and rates of change, so can therapists. Therapists have their own family systems, with their own elements, purpose, interactions, and context. Just because a therapist walks into the therapy room, doesn't mean that they leave their family system behind. The context, competing autonomies, elements, and interactions that are happening in a therapist's family system may create resistance in the therapeutic system – resistance that may be wrongly placed on the clients.

To get good answers, therapists must overcome resistance, both in themselves and in their clients. This isn't an easy task, especially when it comes to our own systems. There have been lots of tips and tricks spelled out by others about how to deal when a client system is resisting. We'll discuss many of those later in this chapter. But to do the work on our own resistance, I only know of one way – self of the therapist work. Specifically, diagnose our own family system.

Systemic Resistance and Self of the Therapist

I've noticed a concerning trend in the family therapy students who complete their master's degree and come to our PhD program – they've never diagnosed their own family system. Often, self of the therapist work that these students are engaged in centers around mindful practices, exercising, or other ways to relax and disconnect. Don't get me wrong, I think that these are good for managing stress, but not so much for dealing with resistance in therapy. To be effective at gathering information to make systemic diagnoses, especially when a system is resisting, we must look first at our own systems. Lucky for you, that's what I'm going to ask you to do.

In family therapy training programs that do ask therapists to look at their own family systems, this is typically done through genograms. To me genograms can be a powerful tool to diagnose a therapist's and a client's family systems. Genograms provide an excellent framework for gathering information about the elements in the family system and the sources of competing autonomy. However, I've found that when students are asked to complete a genogram of their own family, it's often done without much theory. Software has been developed to facilitate genogram creation (e.g., Genopro). This software, while helpful, isn't theory driven. These programs can help you organize information about your family system, but they won't tell you what is important and what isn't. As such, I think it's important to engage in an EPIC evaluation of your family system along with doing a genogram. I think that this is best done before you begin illustrating the genogram. To me, this roots the genogram in theory – something I believe is necessary for it to be effective at helping a therapist diagnose their family. There are many great articles written about doing genograms. My favorites are anything written by Monica McGoldrick. But to accompany these tools, I've provided you with some additional workbook pages in this chapter. I want you to use these workbook pages to create a systemic diagnosis of your own family system. You can use the pages or you can also download them on my website – jacobpriest.com. To use these pages, you're going to have to have completed the *Doing the Work – Questions* section early in this chapter. I want you to use the questions you created in that section to prompt responses about your own family system. I've created space where you can write out your responses to your questions based on your own family system. After you write down this information, I want you to write out a paragraph or two that describes the history, structure, and boundary of your family. I want you to diagnose your family system. Then, I'd encourage you to use your responses and the diagnosis of your family system to create a genogram.

If you are in a family therapy training program, I'd also encourage you to use your questions to ask your fellow students about their family system and have them do the same for you. Not only will this give you good practice using your questions to gather information from another person, but when you talk through these responses out loud, I feel like you sometimes surprise yourself by how you might respond.

If you really want to begin doing this work, I'd hope you'd take this activity outside of the classroom. Use your questions to interview other members of your family system. Based on the information they give you, write a more accurate systemic diagnosis. In my experience, doing this type of self of the therapist work can reduce the amount of resistance a therapist brings to the therapy room.

My Family's Systemic Diagnosis

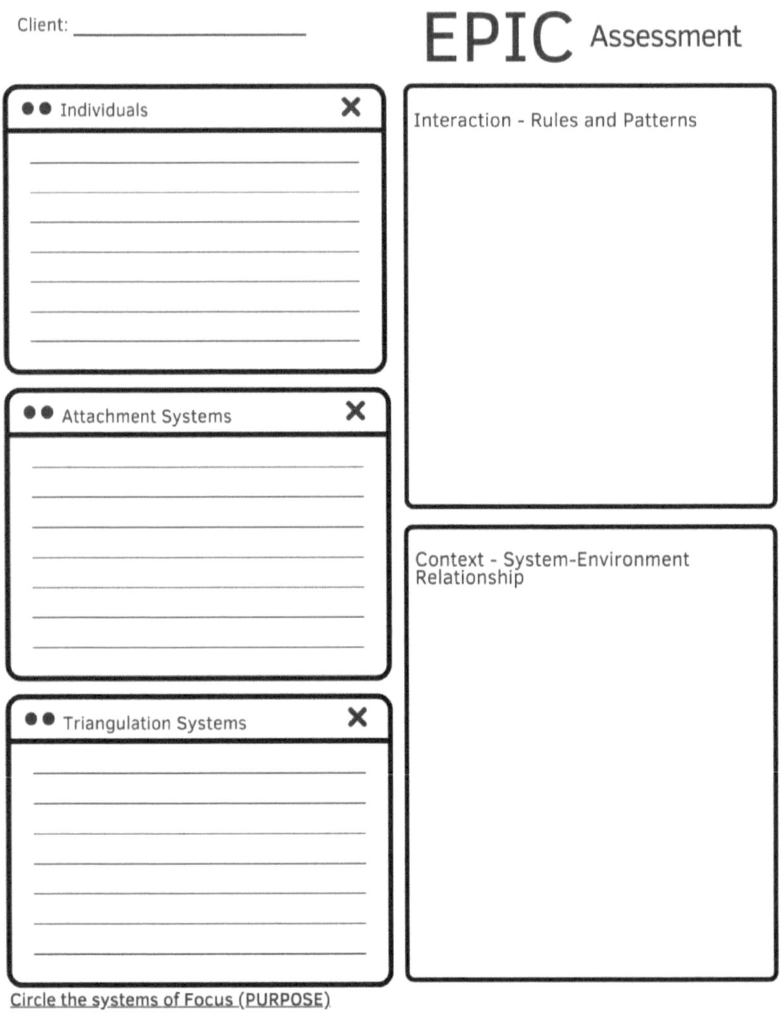

Client: _____

EPIC Assessment

● ● Individuals   ✕

● ● Attachment Systems   ✕

● ● Triangulation Systems   ✕

Circle the systems of Focus (PURPOSE)

Interaction - Rules and Patterns

Context - System-Environment Relationship

Figure 8.1 EPIC assessment sheet

Resistance and Therapeutic Flexibility

Regardless of how much self of the therapist work we do, we are still going to encounter resistance in the clients we work with. When we encounter resistance in a client, often therapists develop ways to try to work around it. A 2010 article published by *Counseling Today* provides a list of nine "quick tips" that therapists can use to manage client

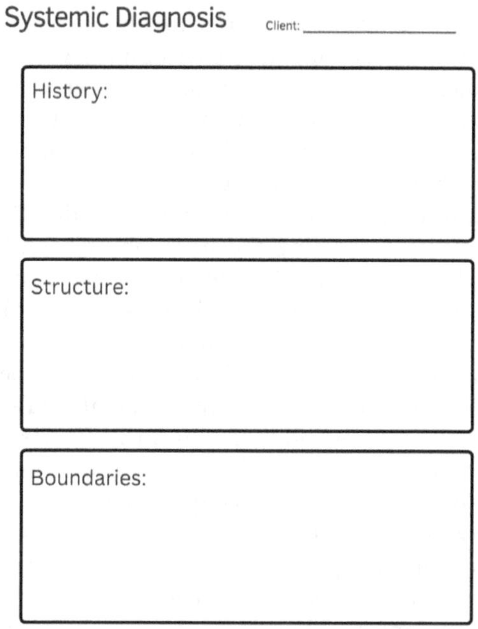

Systemic Diagnosis   Client: _____

History:

Structure:

Boundaries:

Figure 8.2 Systemic diagnosis worksheet

resistance. These include things like "don't collude with client's excuses" and "stay out of an excessive questioning mode." These tips and others can be useful when dealing with resistance – especially in the intervention phase of therapy. However, when it comes to creating a systemic diagnosis, resistance is not something we want to manage; rather, it is something that we can learn from.

I mentioned earlier in this chapter that all systems resist. If the rate of change is too great, systems can lose their autonomy. The interactions that produce a system's autonomy do adapt in response to pressure, but resistance is just a way to manage the exchanges between the structure of the system and its environment. A system would lose its autonomy if it didn't have the capacity to resist. Interactions between elements in a system need to be robust, they need to resist pressure. I think that what frustrates therapists about clients who are resistant is that resistance thwarts intervention. When clients are resistant, they don't want to adapt their autonomy generating process. They don't like intervention that tries to change them. However, if we are diagnosing a system, resistance can provide us with some of the best information regarding a system's history, structure, and boundaries. Resistance can be the path of least resistance to uncovering the purpose, interacting, and context of a system.

When clients are resistant, they are showing you the boundary they use to regulate exchanges with their environment when they are under pressure. The therapist or the therapeutic context is a threat to their autonomy. To deal with the threat, they must activate the processes and interactions that they typically use when dealing with an outside threat. The system may shut down, it may be belligerent, or it may blame other systems. The more we push against the boundary that the structure and history of the system are enacting, the more robust it sometimes becomes. While this may be an issue in the intervention stage of therapy, in the diagnosis stage, it's great information. The tricky part is to get good information about the elements, purpose, interaction, and context of a system; just pushing against a boundary won't work. Clients expect therapists to ask them questions – most people have a general idea of what therapy looks like. Because the question is seen as a threat, to really understand the boundaries, therapists need to be able to gather information about the system in ways other than through questions.

Let me share an example. If you've ever worked with a teenager who doesn't want to be in therapy – especially with their family – they rarely talk. They may not even look at you. The more you ask questions, the more they refuse to answer, shut down, or even get angry. Often, when you do that, the parents might say something like: "This is exactly what happens when I try to talk to them at home." These teens expect questions – their parents ask them questions, their teachers ask them questions – and they know a therapist is going to ask them questions, so they resist. But, we've already found a place of competing autonomy and a rule of interactions in the system. Questions are seen as a threat to the teenager's autonomy, and not answering these questions is seen as a threat to the attachment system of the parent and teen by the parent. The competing autonomy has become the homeostatic pattern of this attachment system – leading the system to be on a disintegrating trajectory. As the therapist, asking questions has given you insight into this important pattern, but it has also shown you that you won't get additional information if you continue in the same pattern. So, what do you do?

When this happens to me, I tend to ask to meet with the teen alone. I start by asking a few questions, and when they don't answer I'll say something like, "Cool. Well, we have like 15 more minutes we need to burn, do you mind just sitting here while I check my email?" Often the teen will muddle something about not caring. After a few minutes of doing this, I'll ask if it's okay if I turn on some music if I work. Again, it's often a muddled response – but teens tend to like music that's very different than what I like. I graduate high school in 2000, and during my college years, I listened to emo music on repeat. To this day, my favorite band is Dashboard Confessional. My wife tells me it can be kind of whiny and annoying – but I think she is totally wrong. When I start playing Dashboard Confessional, the kid will typically pull out their phone or put in headphones. When time is up, I'll tell the kid that they are free to go, but before they do I'll ask something like, "Who were you listening to?" The most common response I get is, "You wouldn't know." My response to this, "Try me."

In my experience after a few times of these types of meetings, the teenager tells me the music they were listening to. If I'm not familiar with it, I'll spend time between our next meeting listening to that band or genre. When they come back, I have the knowledge I need to start a conversation – one that doesn't reinforce a resistant pattern, but also gives me good information. As we talk about music, it circumvents the pattern. Instead of just getting information about the boundary, I can start gleaning information about the purpose, interactions, and context of the system. By shifting the way I try and gather information, I am shifting what information the system will divulge. While we often think the best way to gather information is to ask questions, with certain systems we are going to need other tools to do so.

It may not fit for you to deal with resistance in clients the way I just described. But to make accurate systemic diagnoses, you are going to need to develop your own way of gathering information other than direct questions. One way might be to employ psychometrically validated instruments into your intake paperwork. We have hundreds of questionnaires and assessments that have been developed that can help gather good information about the elements, purpose, interactions, and context of a system. Many of these have had research examine the validity and reliability of these instruments. While there is still a long way to go to make their questionnaires reliable and valid for people from many different contexts, these tools can still be an effective way to gather good information in addition to the questions that you'll ask your clients in the therapy room. If you are looking for a place to start to find measure that might be useful, I recommend checking out the book chapter, *Couple and Family Assessment* by Douglas Snyder (2019) and his colleges. Their work chronicles measures that have had psychometric work done and can help you start to think about why and how you could incorporate them into your practice.

Another way to learn how to gather information without questions, is to become good at seeing rules and patterns. It's sometimes hard to do this with clients, but it can be easier to do this with fictional families. A great resource for finding this is called psychmovies.com. This is a database that lists movies that illustrate psychological concepts. If you go to the "Movie Lists" tab, you'll see a link to one that focuses on "Marital/Family Dynamics." This page contains lists of movies and accompanying descriptions. If you're a family therapy nerd like me, you may want to spend a night watching these movies with a copy of the EPIC assessment sheet and a glass of wine. Practicing this way can not only help you be better at finding the elements, purpose, interactions, and context of these families, but may also be a bit fun.

Finally, to gather good information without asking direct questions, you are going to need to be creative. As such, I've created another worksheet for you – one that just allows you to brainstorm different ideas. If you are in a training program or class when you read this book, I'd encourage you to do this with your fellow classmates. If you don't have anyone to do this with, the exercise can still be useful. It just might be more of a reflection of ways you gathered information from clients without asking questions rather than a brainstorming exercise.

1. What are ways you could learn the elements of a system without asking clients directly?
2. How might you be able to find elements or systems that are competing for autonomy if a couple or family is angry or disengaged?
3. What could you do in the therapy to get the system to show patterns of interactions?
4. How could you learn about the context of a system without asking directly about it?

To accurately make systemic diagnoses, you need to become good at gathering information. Questions are important, but so is the ability to deal with your own and your client's resistance. What I've talked about in this chapter is just the first step. Perfecting the craft of gathering information, doing self of the therapist work, and having therapeutic flexibility in the face of the client's resistance will be something you will refine throughout your career. These things are fundamental to becoming an expert at diagnosing systems. I hope that as you work as a therapist, you not only think about how you ask questions, but also how to gather information without asking questions. What's more, self of the therapist work is key to systemic diagnosis. When you enter a system, you are going to be affected by it. If you haven't systemically diagnosed your own family system, you may be unwittingly assuming that what's going on in your family is going on with your clients. As in the other chapters, I'm going to summarize the main ideas of this one. Hopefully this summary can help you remember to consistently engage in the work of improving your method of asking questions and getting answers.

Recap: Main Ideas and Arguments

1. **Gathering good information means asking good questions.**
    A therapist interview process should be theory driven and slow
    and should reflect the information gathered back to the system.
2. **Resistance is a key component of any family system.** For a sys-
    tem to maintain its autonomy, it must resist. That is the whole
    purpose of the boundary of the system. This boundary regu-
    lates the rate of change and exchanges with the environment. In
    the therapeutic environment, we should expect family systems
    to resist by regulating the exchanges and the rate of change.
3. **Resistance also exists in the therapist's family system.** The con-
    text, competing autonomies, elements, and interactions that
    are happening in a therapist's family system may create resist-
    ance in the therapeutic system – resistance that may be wrongly
    placed on the clients.
4. **Doing self of the therapist work is key to gathering good infor-
    mation.** Therapists have their own family systems, with their
    own elements, purpose, interactions, and context. Just because
    a therapist walks into the therapy room doesn't mean that they
    leave their family system behind. To be effective at gathering
    information to make systemic diagnoses, especially when a sys-
    tem is resisting, we must look first at our own family systems.
5. **Sometimes questions won't get us the information we need.**
    To make accurate systemic diagnoses, you are going to need
    to develop your own way of gathering information other than
    direct questions. One way might be to employ psychometrically
    validated instruments into your intake paperwork. Another
    way to learn how to gather information without asking direct
    questions is to practice seeing rules and patterns by assessing
    fictional families.

Chapter 9

Case Example

Supervision

Gathering good information and making an accurate systemic diagnosis takes practice. Just like any skill, to get good at it, you need to do it over and over. Much of the practice you'll get will be with your own clients in your own therapy room – that's where you'll hone your skills and develop a process that works for you. But I want to help you feel as prepared as possible before you do this with your own clients.

In this example, I want to present what a conversation might look like between me and a supervisor. In this made-up conversation, I'm going to show how I would talk about the EPIC assessment and systemic diagnosis. My goal is to hopefully make the concepts take a bit more shape in your mind and help you think through the systemic diagnostic process. So, the following is a hypothetical conversation between me and my graduate student Kai.

Me: Hey, Kai. Good to see you. What clients do you want to talk about today?

Kai: Well, I have one case in particular that I'm kinda stuck on. I'm trying to really grasp what's going on, but I can't seem to get hold of it.

Me: Ok. So, are you trying to systemically diagnose this family?

Kai: Yeah. I'm trying, but I don't think I'm doing it very well.

Me: Alright, well let's review the important information we need to gather to make a systemic diagnosis. Do you remember what that is?

Kai: Yep. EPIC. Which stands for elements, purpose, interaction, and context. Right?

Me: That's right. To make sure we are clear, let's talk about each one – starting with elements. What are elements and which elements are we looking at?

Kai: Elements are the systems that create the system. They are the things that interact with other things. In the case I'm stuck with, the individual elements include Jenny, the person I'm working with; Jenny's boyfriend, Mateo; Jenny's parents – Karl and Mary; and Jenny's

DOI: 10.4324/9781003295907-12

younger brother Jerry. There are other people we talk about, but these are the main ones.

Me: Great. If these are the individual elements, what are the attachment elements?

Kai: Well, there's the one between Jenny and Mateo; between Jenny and her dad; Jenny and her mom; and Jenny and her brother. But also, the ones between Karl and Mary, between Karl and Jerry, between Mary and Jerry. Mateo also is in attachment systems with Karl, Mary, and Jerry.

Me: Okay, and the triangulation systems?

Kai: Well, umm, Jenny, Mateo, and Karl. Jenny, Mateo, and Mary. Jenny, Jerry, and Karl. Jenny, Jerry, and Mary. Also there's the triangles with Karl, Mary, and Jerry and Karl, Mary, and Mateo. Oh yeah, Mateo, Jenny, and Jerry. Am I missing any?

Me: It's a lot to keep track of, but with these spelled out, can you tell me the next step bit of information we need?

Kai: Well the "p" in EPIC is purpose.

Me: Correct. And what is purpose in systemic diagnosis?

Kai: Purpose is about autonomy. The purpose of every element or system is to maintain autonomy.

Me: Yes. And what is autonomy?

Kai: It's the interactions that serve to generate and maintain the system. And elements can sometimes have places where they compete for autonomy.

Me: Exactly, and what does it mean for elements to have competing autonomy?

Kai: Well, I think it's about the interactions that are occurring in one system, threaten, or put pressure on other systems. Each system wants to keep the same interactions that they are used to. And sometimes that causes problems. Did I get that right?

Me: Yes, and maybe I'd just add a bit more too. Elements are a part of multiple systems and so the competing autonomy between systems not only puts pressure on or threatens other systems but also can make adaptation different even in the short or long term.

Kai: Oh yeah, and this is for sure happening with Jenny.

Me: Say more about that. What are the systems that Jenny is in that seem to be competing for autonomy?

Kai: Well, for sure the attachment system between her and her dad. I mean that was the impetus for her coming to therapy. They aren't getting along. Her dad doesn't really accept her or her relationship with Mateo.

Me: Okay, so we aren't just talking about competing autonomy in the attachment system between Jenny and Karl, but also in the Jenny-Karl-Mateo triangle.

Kai: Yes.

Me: Okay, so any other systems where elements are competing for autonomy?

Kai: Well, probably in Jenny's parents' attachment system; when we talk about her dad we talk a lot about her parents' relationship and how she wants her relationship to be very different than her parents.

Me: Okay, any other systems that Jenny is a part of that might be important?

Kai: Well, it's not just conflict right?

Me: Right.

Kai: So, I would also say the system of Jenny, Mateo, and Jerry. There isn't any conflict there, but Jenny is always talking about how she wants Mateo and Jerry to be better friends.

Me: Great, so the systems we want to focus our attention on are the Jenny-Mateo-Karl triangle and the attachment and individual systems within it, the Jenny-Karl-Mary triangle and those attachment and individual systems, and the Jenny-Mateo-Jerry triangle and those attachment and individual systems.

Kai: That seems right to me.

Me: Okay, what comes next?

Kai: We need to track interactions in these systems. It's the "i" in EPIC.

Me: That's right. How do we do that?

Kai: We look for patterns or rules within these systems.

Me: Yes, but before we jump there, we need to remember what creates interaction in a family system. Do you remember the three processes that give rise to interactions?

Kai: I think so . . . threat-response, belonging, and, uh, individuality?

Me: Yes. Do you remember what those are or what type of interactions they create?

Kai: Well, threat-response is about changes in the environment or new information. It's what elements in a system do when something happens within or outside of the system that the system must accommodate.

Me: Exactly. And the other two?

Kai: Well, individually processes is any interaction that tries to maintain the autonomy of the different elements within the system, and belonging processes are the interactions that keep the elements together.

Me: And what are the main types of rules that a family system has? What ones are we going to make sure and assess for?

Kai: We want to think about their homeostasis rule?

Me: Good. What do homeostasis rules do?

Kai: They are all about the stability of the system; what keeps it going internally. The others are about flexibility and boundaries.

Me: That's right. Flexibility rules do what?

Kai: Well, they tell us how a family responds to stress or pressure.

Me: And boundaries?

Kai: Those are about how the family responds or reacts to their environment.

Me: Great. So let's talk about the first attachment system you brought – Jenny's relationship with her dad. What patterns or rules do you see in that system?

Kai: I think this is where I'm stuck. Jenny is super anxious, so the first couple of times I met with her, she just threw lots of information at me and I felt a bit overwhelmed.

Me: Okay, well let's start with Jenny – she's an important element in this system. I know she threw a lot at you but as you look back on what you talked about with her, do you recognize any themes or patterns?

Kai: What I remember her saying the most is "not being enough." Lots of her anxiety is about being rejected or people getting to know the real her and her not liking it. She's worried about not being enough.

Me: So, if this is the story she's telling you, what processes are going on inside of her that are part of this pattern?

Kai: Her threat-response processes are elevated. She's always looking for signs that people are saying that she is not enough. Like, she seems to feel that everywhere – especially when she sees her dad.

Me: Say more about how it plays out with her dad – in that attachment system.

Kai: Ok, well, she feels like she is constantly letting her dad down, that she wants him to accept her but that she never gets what she needs from him. He doesn't show up for her the way she wants.

Me: When she's with her dad, when they interact, what happens?

Kai: Jenny would describe it as her reaching out – trying to get him to talk – and her dad just pulling back – ignoring her or not really paying attention.

Me: And when her dad does this, what does Jenny do?

Kai: She tries harder. She pushes until finally she gives up.

Me: And what does giving up on her dad look like?

Kai: She stops trying to connect with him for a while. She may complain to her mom and Mateo about it, but she just stops.

Me: Does her dad eventually reach out? Does he try to get the interaction going again?

Kai: Yeah. Eventually, he gives her something – Jenny guesses it comes from pressure from her mom – and then Jenny jumps right back in.

Me: So, this pattern you're describing, has it always been like this? Has it changed or gotten more apparent recently?

Kai: I think Jenny would say it's always been like this. Her dad has always been distant, and she's had to pursue him. But I would think that it's gotten more problematic since Jenny started dating Mateo.

Me: Okay. Before we jump to the triangle, I want to solidify the pattern in the Jenny-Karl system. This seems like a pattern that allows that system to maintain its autonomy. It almost seems like the baseline or homeostatic pattern. Like, without this pattern, there is no interaction.

Kai: I think that's a fair assessment. It has been their interaction pattern forever. Karl seems pretty distant, and Jenny pushes for that connection. This is pretty much what keeps their system going. I don't think they know how to interact any other way.

Me: Okay, so let's talk about how Mateo and Jenny's relationship and the creation of the Jenny-Mateo-Karl triangle.

Kai: Well, Jenny and Mateo met their senior year of college – about two years ago. After college they decided to get a place together – they've been living together about a year.

Me: How would you or how does Jenny describe their relationship?

Kai: Jenny would say it's really great. She doesn't make this comparison, but they way she describes Mateo is like the complete opposite of her dad. Mateo is attentive and affectionate. He likes to communicate.

Me: And Jenny feels comfortable and happy in this relationship?

Kai: She does. But she also doesn't completely trust it. Mateo would want to propose to her and get married, but she's not ready for it. She says she loves Mateo but she's not in the place where he's at.

Me: How would you describe their interaction. What are the rules or patterns of their attachment system?

Kai: It's kind of similar to Jenny and her dad's, but in the opposite direction. Mateo pushes to connect, Jenny pulls aways. Mateo then asks Jenny about where she is at and if she wants to stay in this relationship – his version of pulling back, and then Jenny usually engages and connects with him and everything is great for a while. Then Jenny gets distant and Mateo pushes for more connection.

Me: And has this been a pattern that has been present in their relationship since the start?

Kai: I think so. Jenny says that Mateo very much pursued her. When they first met, he was pretty assertive and Jenny really liked feeling wanted.

Me: Okay, so would you say that this pattern is the interaction that maintains Jenny and Mateo's system? Is this their homeostasis?

Kai: Yes. I think so.

Me: Let's expand it out and talk about these rules and how they shape the Jenny-Karl-Mateo triangle. Do you think these patterns are connected?

Kai: Totally. It seems like when Jenny is most concentrated on getting close with her dad, that's when she gets distant from Mateo. When Mateo pushes for more connection, it almost seems like Jenny pushes her dad more. When Mateo finally starts to bring up concerns with Jenny, this is when Jenny gives up with her dad and focuses on her relationship with Mateo. After that happens for a while, she gets a message from her dad and she starts to focus on that relationship. And then the interactions plays out over and over.

Me: Makes sense that Jenny is anxious. These attachments and this triangle really need Jenny's anxiety to keep the patterns going.

Kai: That's for sure.

Me: I know we have a few other elements and systems to talk through, but I want to make sure we are clear about this triangle. Is there any important context that we should be talking about to better understand these rules and patterns.

Kai: Context? Yes, the "c" in EPIC.

Me: Yep. Do you remember what we mean by context in systemic diagnosis?

Kai: Yes. Context is the "why" of the system. It is the history and development of a system. It's what makes the rules and patterns make sense.

Me: Exactly. So what are important contexts of these attachment and triangle systems? What has happened in the past? How do these systems interact with their social environment? Why don't we start with the important context of the Jenny-Karl system?

Kai: Yes, there is some important context there. Karl grew up in poverty. He started working when he was really young and hasn't stopped. He's been really successful in his career, but he's in his 60s now and Jenny says that she doesn't see him retiring or slowing down. She thinks that he uses work as an excuse to be so distant.

Me: And what does Jenny's dad think?

Kai: When Jenny complains to Karl or when she tries to connect, he always deflects by telling her all the things he's paid for. He'll say things like, "you wouldn't have that fancy degree, if I didn't work so hard."

Me: You mean her college degree?

Kai: Yeah, Jenny has a degree in art history – her dad paid for her to go to college. He wanted her to go to the state school, but Jenny had her heart set on a liberal arts college. Her dad is pretty conservative, and Jenny got more liberal when she went to school. Part of what fuels the distance in their relationship is their political ideology – or at least that's what Jenny would say.

Me: So, Karl comes from poverty and Jenny has always had a pretty stable financial situation?

Kai: Yeah. She's never really had to worry about it. Even now, when things get financially tight, her dad will give her money. Well, Jenny will let her mom know and then her dad sends her a check. That's sometimes how they start talking again.

Me: Okay. And what about Mateo. What's the important context about him?

Kai: Mateo is a Dreamer – his parents came to the States when he was really young. Jenny says that Karl sometimes implies that he thinks that Mateo just wants to marry Jenny for her money and to get citizenship.

Me: That must be really hurtful for Mateo.

Kai: Yeah, he has really tried to connect with Karl, but Karl can be pretty mean.

Me: And Karl sometimes helps them financially?

Kai: Yeah, Jenny says Mateo hates asking her dad for money. But Jenny does it anyway, especially when things are tight. Mateo had a great job, but the company got bought out and so he lost his job. He got severance for a bit, but still didn't have another job when that ran out. They had to get some help from Karl until Mateo was employed again.

Me: How do you think all of this context influences the patterns in the attachment and in the triangle?

Kai: Let's see. Mateo feels like the outsider in the triangle – something that Jenny says he's felt at times throughout his life. Karl has the power – at least the financial power – that allows him to try and control the patterns. He gets to decide whether to help or not, and this can give him cover for the way he acts in his relationships. Jenny feels powerless except for when she withdraws from either Mateo or her dad. When she does this, that's when she can get what she wants or feel a sense of control for a little while. Her anxiety is better when she does this, but spikes right back up when the pattern plays out.

Me: So, Jenny's threat-response processes are really active in this triangle in part because of the context. She is always at risk of losing the connection in her attachment systems? But the pattern in the triangle needs her to have these over-active threat-response processes?

Kai: Right. Jenny is constantly trying to navigate belonging in one attachment system at the expense of the other attachment system. These two systems really are competing for autonomy. But the triangulation system exists only because of this. Jenny stays connected to both her dad and Mateo through these patterns. Mateo and Karl need to be in conflict, or the pattern doesn't really play out in either attachment system.

Me: In other words, the homeostatic rules that are created need Jenny to be anxious. If she stops being anxious and at times over functioning for her dad, and under functioning with Mateo, the attachment systems would lose their autonomy?

Kai: I think that's right. And the triangle needs this competition. It would lose its autonomy if there wasn't this pressure for Jenny to go back and forth.

Me: Okay, but what about the flexibility rules? What happens to this pattern when it's under stress? Which way does it polarize?

Kai: Oh, it's super rigid. Everyone does take the same role when things are stressed. That has been the case since Jenny was young.

Me: Say more about that.

Kai: Jenny would say that her dad was very strict growing up. If there were ever stress at work, the same pattern would play out, it would just play out louder and longer.

Me: Karl would get angry?

Kai: Yes. Any thought that he could lose his financial security would send him into a panic. Instead of just asking for help, he'd get angry and pull away. Everyone knew when dad "needed space," as Jenny would say.

Me: So the structure of the family is pretty rigid?

Kai: Yes, regardless of the stress, it seems that Karl, Jenny, and Jenny's mom would do the same thing.

Me: So, you're talking about the history of how the system has adapted in the past. Instead of generating lots of ways to respond to stress, does the family just get stuck and intensify its patterns?

Kai: Yes, the way they've adapted, or not I guess, in the past has led them to be super . . . what's the word . . . calcified.

Me: Okay. It sounds like we have a clear grasp on the systems that are competing, the structure of the system, and about the history and context. Should we try to use this information to make a systemic diagnosis?

Kai: Yeah, I think that would be helpful.

Me: Great, let's start with a summary of the history. What are the important points in their history that have led them to the structure they have today? What are important messages they've adopted from their social systems?

Kai: I think the structure of the system has been shaped by the social systems they have been embedded in. The calcification and polarization of their structure is shaped by the financial power and narratives of gender and race in the social systems they inhabit. Karl has been told that good husbands and fathers provide, Jenny that it is her responsibility as a woman to be responsible for connection, and the limited access to resources that encumber Mateo's ability to work and meet Karl's expectation of a good partner.

Me: Yes. I'd agree. So, summarize what their structure is now.

Kai: Mateo and Jenny's attachment system replicates the pattern she learned with her father, but in it her part is reversed – she pulls away from Mateo, while Mateo pursues her. This pattern has also been calcifying since Mateo lost his job and Jenny asked her father for financial help. When that happened, the pattern in the Jenny-Mateo-Karl triangle was solidified. Mateo began over functioning to maintain his connection with Jenny, while Jenny would float between being distant with her father and distant with Mateo. When she is distant from her father, Karl criticizes Mateo and Jenny, pushing her closer to Mateo, but when she feels overwhelmed by the closeness with Mateo, she pulls away and often asks her father for more financial support. This leads her father to ramp up his criticism of Mateo, especially his status as an immigrant, reducing any flexibility in the system, but eventually leading to renewed closeness with Mateo and cutoff for a few weeks from her father.

Me: Great description. So what about the boundary?

Kai: Well, any outside pressures seem to overwhelm the system, so it does the same thing but just more intensely. When Mateo lost his job, Jenny got closer to her father by asking for help and pulled away from Mateo. This has also made Jenny be constantly scanning for threats within and outside the system. The boundary is such that any pressure seems to amplify their problematic patterns.

Me: That seems clear to me. Does that help you feel less stuck with Jenny?

Kai: I think so. I feel like this has helped me understanding the patterns and what needs to shift. And I think that it also tells me why it's been so hard for Jenny to reduce her anxiety. These systems are easily overwhelmed by pressure and the patterns just get so stuck.

Conversations about systemic diagnosis and supervision are typically more complicated than what I've presented here. The nice thing about creating my own conversations is that I can have them play out exactly as I want. But I do hope this gives you an idea of the process of gathering information and making a systemic diagnosis. In the next chapters, I'm going to just present that content and have you reflect and answer questions.

Chapter 10

Systemic Diagnosis in the Therapy Room

One of my earliest mentors, Randy Chatelain, used to call his therapy room the "emergency room of relationships." When couples would come to see him, it often wasn't for a check-up, it was typically to try to save a relationship that was close to dead or dying. Now that I've been practicing for nearly 15 years, I understand what he means. When couples come to therapy, their relationships typically aren't in good shape. Often, they are angry, shut down, or threatening divorce. When this is the case, it can make gathering information to make a systemic diagnosis difficult. It can be easy to want to intervene to try and save the relationship. But unlike the actual emergency room, trying to intervene immediately can lead to intervention that may hurt rather than help a system. I think that when a system is in real distress, taking the extra time to assess the system to make a systemic diagnosis is the best way to help a couple's relationship.

Let me show you what I mean. The second case example we are going to use is of a couple I'll call Ang and Joel. Ang and Joel have been married for five years, they have a 2-year-old son and as you'll see, they are both hurt, angry, and scared of losing their relationship. In these circumstances, it can be hard to stay focused on gathering information. But as you'll see, gathering information can be tricky when a system feels under immense pressure. As such, I've structured this case study to focus on each aspect of the EPIC assessment. At the end of the dialogue, I'm going to present you with some questions, and I want you to make your own systemic diagnosis. I'll give you space to do so, and if you want, you can compare yours to what others have written by going to my website (jacobpriest.com). There, I have uploaded examples of systemic diagnoses of others who have been presented this case study.

Me: Thanks to both of you for coming here today. I wanted to start out by talking about what brought you to therapy and what you hope to get out of it.
Ang: Well, you tell him.
Joel: What? This was your idea.

DOI: 10.4324/9781003295907-13

Ang: This was *my* idea? God, seriously! You're going to make me tell him?

Joel: Don't jump down my throat, geez.

Ang: Fine. Joel has been messaging his ex.

Joel: And how do you know that? You hacked into my account, right?

Ang: That is so not the point.

Joel: What did the messages say? I wasn't cheating or anything, we didn't even meet up.

Ang: But you lied about it! I asked you point blank if you'd been talking to her, and you told me you hadn't. Then I found these messages.

Joel: You found the messages!? And what did the messages say? Huh? What did they say?

Ang: I don't care about that. I care that you lied.

Joel: When? When did I lie? You asked if I had seen her, and I told you the truth.

Ang: You didn't lie? Really? You didn't? I don't fucking believe this. You are so full of shit. You didn't lie. Okay. Why are we even here then?

Joel: I don't know. This was your idea.

Me: I'm going to jump in and slow us down a little. Sounds like we have a lot to unpack, and I want to make sure that I get all of the important information. Ang, is it okay if I start with you?

Ang: Yeah, that's fine.

Me: Okay, back me up a bit. You said you found messages from Joel to an ex. How long ago was this?

Ang: You mean this time or when it happened before?

Joel: Really? You're gonna bring . . .

Me: Hey, Joel, I'm going to check back with you, I promise. I just need you to hold tight for a bit while I chat with Ang and then I'm going to come back to you, okay?

Joel: Yeah, sure, okay.

Me: Thanks. Okay, so Ang, let's just focus on what happened recently. Can you walk me through that timeline?

Ang: Sure. So, it was probably like a month or so ago. Joel is always on his phone, but I just felt something was up – he was on his phone more than usual. I figured that something was going on. When he went to put Jack to bed, I grabbed his phone and that's when I saw all of the messages.

Me: Who's Jack?

Ang: Our son. He's 2.

Me: And you do you have other kids or just Jack?

Ang: Just Jack.

Me: Okay, so Joel puts Jack to bed, and you check his phone and what do you see?

Joel: Can I . . .

Me: Hold on just a second, okay?

Ang: I saw like so many messages from her. Like they had been talking for like two weeks.

Joel: It wasn't that long.

Ang: I don't care, whatever. But there were a ton of messages. They had been talking a lot.

Me: After you saw the messages, then what happened?

Ang: He came up from putting Jack to bed, and I asked him if he'd been talking to Becky.

Me: Becky is the ex?

Ang: Yes. And he said that he hadn't. He straight up lied to my face. And then I showed him his phone.

Me: And what did you say to him?

Ang: I threw the phone at him and told him to fuck off.

Me: Did you leave the room? Or what did you do?

Ang: I left. I got in the car and just fucking drove. I was so fucking mad. I couldn't believe he was lying again about her.

Me: About Becky?

Ang: Yes. He did this before, when we were engaged. Like two months before our wedding, he did the exact same thing.

Joel: No, it wasn't the same thing. I mean come on. Can I jump in?

Me: Sure. Why don't you tell me what you remember about that night?

Joel: I had been messaging Becky, but it was just about her parents. When we dated, I was really close to her mom and her mom has been having some health stuff recently, so I just checked in. That's all.

Ang: Oh, uh-huh, sure. Just checked in. You were close to her mom? Since when?

Joel: Can I talk? God, you never let me talk. All I did was talk about her mom and we caught up a bit.

Ang: Caught up a bit? After you promised me you'd never talk with her again after the first time!

Me: Let's talk more about that. Joel, what happened the first time? Ang said this was two months before your wedding? How long have you been married?

Joel: Just over five years. Yeah, so when we were engaged, I was chatting with Becky. We talked about it, and I thought we had worked through it, but I guess not.

Ang: Talked about it? We didn't talk about it. I basically broke up with you and you begged me to come back.

Joel: I didn't beg.

Ang: Okay, whatever, I don't care. But you almost blew up everything in our relationship – for her – and here you are doing it again.

Joel: This is different.

Ang: How? How is it different?

Joel: I'm not blowing up our relationship. We were just talking.

Ang: Sure. You expect me to believe that you were just talking?

Me: I know this is hard to rehash this stuff, but if we are going to work together I'm going to need to make sure I'm getting what's going on with you two. Let me know if I'm getting it. Right before you got married, Joel was talking with Becky. That led to a big argument between you two where you almost broke up, but you got back together and you've been married for five years and Jack is now 2. And then about a month ago you had another argument because of these new messages between Joel and Becky? Am I missing anything so far?

Joel: Why don't you tell him where you drove that night? Where'd you go?

Ang: I went to my sister's house.

Joel: Like you always do.

Ang: Where else am I supposed to go?

Joel: You could talk to me.

Ang: So, you can lie some more?

Me: Hang on a second. Ang, what's your sister's name? Is she older, younger? Does she live close to you?

Ang: Her name is Lin. She's my older sister, she is just like 20 months older than I am. She lives like an hour away. We've always been super close. She's like my best friend.

Joel: You tell her everything – no wonder she hates me.

Ang: She doesn't hate you. And, when you lie, I tell her that you lie.

Me: Okay. So, your sister, Lin, lives about an hour away. That night you drove to her house. How long did you stay there?

Ang: A few hours. We got in a fight, and I left around 8 but I didn't get back until like 3 in the morning.

Me: And Joel, what were you doing?

Joel: Trying to get her on the phone. I called her like 20 times, but she never answered. Jack woke up crying because of our fight but after he went back to sleep, I just assumed she went to her sister's house, so I went to bed.

Me: Joel, do you have anyone that you talk to about these types of things? Is there anyone that you have like Ang has Lin?

Joel: Not really.

Ang: That's not true. I know exactly who you are telling.

Joel: Who?

Ang: I guarantee that if you showed me your text messages right now to John, he'd know all about what's going on.

Joel: That's different.

Ang: How? How is that different?

Joel: I'm just blowing off steam to John. He knows that it's not serious.

Ang: Okay then, show me.

Joel: What?

Ang: Show me what you wrote to John.

Joel: God. Here we go again. I'm always the bad guy.

Me: Hold on a second. Who's John?

Joel: John is my best friend. I've known him since like fourth grade.

Me: And is this someone that you would vent to when you and Ang get in an argument?

Joel: Sure. You know, I'd say things to him, but he knows it's not serious.

Me: Ang, it sounds like you have concerns about what Joel says to John?

Ang: Yeah. I think they talk shit about me on those messages and that's why he won't let me see them.

Me: Okay, I know there is a lot going on, but I want to make sure I know all the people involved before we dive too deep into this. Is there anyone else that either of you talk to or use for support when things get stressful? Are there any other important people that I should know about? Other family members or friends I should be aware of?

Joel: Her parents.

Ang: My parents?!? We should talk about your parents.

Joel: What? How they are helpful and supportive?

Ang: Really? Your parents? Who never wanted us to be together in the first place?

Joel: That's bullshit. You know that they love you.

Me: Can I jump in here? Ang, tell me a bit about your parents. Do they live close to you?

Ang: Kinda. They are about three hours away. But I'm not as close to them as I am to my sister.

Me: What do you mean?

Ang: My parents immigrated from Hong Kong when I was really young. They have a totally different world view, and I get frustrated with them because they want me to be someone I'm not.

Me: How so?

Ang: They are religious, and I'm not really anymore. They are still super connected to Hong Kong and their community, and I'm not. I've only been there once, and I couldn't really communicate with my relatives.

Me: So they're not really close to you, are they close to Jack? Do you feel like they support you and Joel?

Ang: They wanted me to marry someone from our culture – if not from Hong Kong at least someone who goes to the same church. And that's not Joel. They love being grandparents – this is their first grandkid, and they help out a lot when they can. We are just so different, it's hard. I mean, they support us way more than Joel's parents.

Me: Hold up, Ang, I want to ask Joel about that. Joel, Ang thinks that your parents aren't supportive of her or of your relationship. Do you agree?

Joel: No. That's ridiculous.

Me: How come?

Joel: The only reason she would think that is because her parents didn't like me. They just came to my defense.

Ang: That's not true. God, can you just . . .

Me: Okay, let's pull back again. It sounds like there are some relationships beside just you two where there is lots of stress. I want to make sure I know how they affect you. So let me know if I'm missing something. Okay?

Ang: Okay.

Joel: Yeah.

Me: There seems to be a history of tension between your relationship and one or both of your sets of parents. You may disagree on the details, but at certain points you've both felt that the other person's parents haven't been supportive? Is that fair?

Joel: Yeah.

Ang: Not supportive is hardly what they've been. They wanted Joel to end up with Becky. They always have.

Joel: That's not true. God, they said something one time and you've never let it go. I should have never told you that.

Ang: So you think it's just better to keep things from me? Got it.

Joel: That's not what I meant. Geez . . .

Me: Okay, okay. We'll explore that more as we work together but I want to be clear about these other relationships too. Ang you feel close to your sister, and Joel feels like your sister doesn't support him. Joel, you are close to John, but Ange worries that John doesn't respect her. Am I missing anything?

Ang: Don't forget Becky.

Joel: Jesus Christ – she's not important.

Ang: But her mom is?

Me: Hang on a bit. Is this type of interaction the one you both just had what happens at home? You've both done it a few times now, but I'm wondering if it's a pattern for you?

Joel: What do you mean?

Me: Joel, you seem like you felt attacked right there and do you notice what you do when you feel attacked?

Ang: Uh, he lies then pretends . . .

Me: Hold on a second, Ang, I'll come to you in a bit. Joel, it seems to me that you get defensive when you feel attacked. Is that right?

Joel: Yes, I guess.

Me: And what do you do when you get defensive?

Joel: I don't know.

Me: You put up a wall. You push Ang away. Do you see that?

Joel: Kinda. I don't know. I think that she's really the one that makes these things an issue.

Me: Ang, do you ever sense Joel getting defensive? What goes on for you when you see him getting defensive?

Ang: I think he's hiding something. I feel like if he were honest, he wouldn't have to hide things.

Me: So, when Joel gets defensive, you assume he's trying to hide something? So, what do you do?

Ang: I try and figure it out.

Me: And how do you do that?

Ang: I'll ask him straight up and he'll mumble or say something stupid, so I'll have to find it myself.

Joel: You mean snoop.

Ang: I wouldn't snoop if you were honest.

Me: See here it is again – attack-defend; attack-defend. Do this happen around other things?

Ang: I mean now I don't trust him with anything. He's done so much to betray my trust that I don't know if I can ever trust him.

Joel: Trust me? Anytime I try to connect with you, you're the one that pushes me away.

Ang: Sex isn't connection. That's about you, not about me.

Joel: Well, maybe if you didn't reject it all the time . . .

Ang: What you want me to fuck you? I can't fucking stand you.

Joel: God, this is pointless. Do you see what she does? You say I attack? She is the crazy one.

Me: Let me step in here. This is how I see it. It does seem to me that you all attack and defend – especially when things get heated. But it's almost as if, once things get too heated, that's when you turn to other people – like John or Lin.

Ang: I mean, what else am I supposed to do? He doesn't care. He doesn't listen. I'd be totally alone if it wasn't for her.

Joel: So that's okay, but me talking to John isn't? How is that fair?

Ang: Well, then show me what you say to John. Show what you said to him after I left that night.

Joel: Are you going to tell me what Lin said? Huh? I didn't think so. Maybe I should give your parents what they want and leave.

Ang: That's not what they want. They want us together. That's part of the reason I stuck it out. I'm already a disappointment to them. I'm not the perfect son like you are.

Joel: My parents don't think I'm perfect.

Ang: But Becky is?

Me: Alright. Alright, let's take a breath here. I know talking about this stuff is difficult. I want to help you sort through it all, but I need to be clear about what's going on. Joel, can you tell me a bit about your parents?

Joel: Yeah, we're pretty close. I mean my mom and I are. My dad has always been there but not really involved.

Me: What do you mean he's there but not involved?

Joel: Well, I have a sis . . . I mean brother who came out as trans a few years ago. My dad reacted poorly, but I came to my brother's defense and got my dad to shut up. I doubt he's okay with it, but he doesn't say anything about it anymore.

Me: Are you and your brother close? What's your brother's name?

Joel: Taylor. He moved a while back, so I don't see him very often. We weren't ever super close, but he's been more distant since the fight with my dad.

Me: But you and your mom are close?

Ang: She *loves* Becky.

Joel: Becky and I grew up together. My mom said things when Ang and I first started dating like she thought Becky and I would always end up together, but that doesn't mean she doesn't like Ang. I should have never told you that.

Ang: Yeah, just keep more stuff from me. Great.

Joel: You won't tell me what your sister says about me, so I don't want to hear it okay. You don't get what my family is like.

Me: What do you mean by that, Joel?

Joel: My dad cheated on my mom so many times. He used to try and hide it, but we all knew. I'm not close to him because I can't trust him. She thinks I'm just like my dad. She just wants me to cheat so she can leave me.

Ang: That's not true. You always assume things about me that aren't true.

I'm going to stop the conversation there. I think that there is much more to explore regarding the purpose, interactions, and context of this family system, but I do think there is enough information to begin the process. You may need to extrapolate a bit beyond what was presented to make a systemic diagnosis, but I think that can be a useful exercise. Finding the holes or places that still need to be explored and making hypotheses about what might be there can help you ask the right questions. So, to help you make a systemic diagnosis from this dialogue I want you to answer the following questions. After you answer these questions, I want you to write out an initial systemic diagnosis. Like I said at the beginning of the chapter, if you want to see what others have done, head over to my website – jacobpriest.com – and compare what you wrote to what others have.

Chapter 11

AI Generated Examples

One of my least favorite parts of writing this book was trying to generate case examples. I often feel like creating these examples can be useful but also problematic. The examples I've created throughout this book all come from my head. They reflect my experience, my training, and the clients I've worked with. They are biased because of that. What's more, I'm not a playwright. My training has never been on creating dialogue that is interesting – it's been about therapy, theory, and diagnosis. I've tried to do the best job I could to illustrate the concepts I've presented through dialogue. I guess you'll have to judge whether you feel like I've succeeded.

I'm also hesitant to use real dialogue of real clients. It's common practice in many of these books to get permission from clients to share their stories. The authors will change their names and other identifying information, but they will still share details of important conversations they have had with clients. I'm sure many of my clients would have given me permission to share their stories if I asked. But I didn't want to do that either. To me, I want my clients' stories to be their stories. Even if no one could ever identify them, they could identify themselves in my writing. Because of how vulnerable people get in therapy, I don't want them to see me using their stories for my gain. That, to me, just doesn't sit right.

Thankfully for me there are new tools that can help create the examples I need and give you the practice that I think is important. As I'm writing this, ChatGPT has just been released and Microsoft has just announced the infusion of ChatGPT into their search engine Bing. By the time this book is released, it may be that the models that are used to build the artificial intelligence behind ChatGPT have grown exponentially. If AI becomes the powerful tool that many have predicted it will become, it may be that therapists in training will be able to pull up an AI generated client and can practice skills like systemic diagnosis. I can envision a world where therapists accrue their hours for graduation and licensure not just from interfacing with humans but also from AI generated clients.

DOI: 10.4324/9781003295907-14

Many professions currently do this – pilots spend hours in simulators – and it wouldn't surprise me if that became common practice for family therapists.

It may be that AI will become so powerful that it will have the ability to make systemic diagnoses and do systemic interventions better than human therapists. I think we are a long way off from that, if we ever get there at all. But I do think that therapists should think about how AI can help train and evaluate therapists.

Right now, AI isn't that powerful. But it can still be helpful. You can ask ChatGPT to create dialogue of a family or couple in therapy and it will generate it. You can ask it to create dialogue of couples fighting about money, families arguing over inheritance, or a mother and daughter-in-law disagreeing about parenting. And as you'll see in this chapter, I've done just that. To me the examples that ChatGPT generated aren't amazing – they're like some of the dialogue I've written. But I wanted to give you multiple jumping off points that you can use to think through the process of systemic diagnosis. I wanted to give you some snippets of dialogue and have you build out the rest with your own dialogue, questions, and experiences. While AI and ChatGPT may be powerful tools in the future, as currently constituted, I don't think we should be using it anymore than to just help us generate ideas to practice.

All the dialogue I present in this chapter is AI generated. The questions that follow these snippets of dialogue are my own. My goal in combining these two is to give you the practice you need to take systemic diagnosis into your therapy room. I also wanted to show how AI and other tools can be used currently and potentially could more fully hone your systemic diagnosis skills in the future.

Example #1: A Couple Disagreeing About Finances

Person 1: We need to talk about our finances. We're spending too much money on things we don't need.

Person 2: What are you talking about? I don't think we're spending too much.

Person 1: Have you looked at our bank statement? We spent $500 on eating out last month.

Person 2: Well, we deserve to treat ourselves once in a while.

Person 1: That's not the point. We need to be mindful of our spending if we want to reach our financial goals.

Person 2: I don't see why you're making such a big deal about this. It's just $500.

Person 1: It's not just about the $500. It's about making smart choices with our money. We need to start being more responsible.

Person 2: I'm sick of always having to watch every penny we spend. Can't we just enjoy our money for once?

Person 1: Of course we can, but we need to do it within reason. We need to prioritize our expenses and make sure we're putting our money towards things that matter to us.

1. How might this dialogue reflect the homeostasis or flexibility rules of this couple? What additional questions might you ask to see if this pattern has calcified or polarized?
2. If this couple came to therapy with this as one of their main concerns, what questions would you ask about the history or context of the couple? Why would you ask these questions?
3. What would you ask to explore if the conflict is related to other elements or systems in this couple's family? Why would that be important?
4. If you were to write the next few lines of dialogue, how would you do it to demonstrate that this couple is on a disintegrating trajectory? How would it be different if they were on a thriving trajectory?

Example #2: A Daughter-In-Law and Mother-In-Law Disagree About Parenting

Daughter-in-Law: I just can't take it anymore. Every time I try to do something my way, you criticize me and undermine my decisions.

Mother-in-Law: I'm just trying to help. I have more experience in these things.

Daughter-in-Law: I know, but it feels like you're not respecting me as a wife to your son and a mother to your grandchildren.

Mother-in-Law: I do respect you, but I can't just sit back and watch you make mistakes. You're not doing things the right way.

Daughter-in-Law: The right way according to whom? I have my own way of doing things and I think it's working just fine.

Mother-in-Law: Well, I disagree. You don't have the same life experience and knowledge that I do. I just want to make sure you're doing what's best for the family.

Daughter-in-Law: I understand that, but it's not about what's best for the family. It's about what's best for me and my relationship with my husband and children. You need to trust that I have their best interests at heart.

1. If this is one source of competing autonomy or conflict, how would you assess other sources? How would you ask about elements? How would you use your questions about elements to assess for purpose of these elements and the systems they create?

2. What do you assume is the history and context of this conversation? What could you ask to verify that?

3. If you were to watch this pattern play out, how would you assume it would? What do you think would be the next steps if this system were on a disintegrating trajectory? What would happen next if this system were on a thriving trajectory?

Example #3: Parents and A Son Disagreeing About Curfew

Mother: We need to talk to you about your curfew.

Son: What's the problem?

Father: The problem is that you're not respecting the rules we've set for you. Your curfew is 10pm and yet you're coming home much later than that.

Son: I know, but I was hanging out with my friends and the time got away from me.

Mother: We understand that you want to spend time with your friends, but you need to be responsible and follow the rules we've set for your safety.

Son: I know, but I'm almost 18. Don't you think it's time to loosen the rules a bit?

Father: No, it's not time to loosen the rules. You're still living under our roof and following our rules.

1. What attachment systems are present in the conversation? How do these attachment systems form a triangulation system?

2. How do you think this interaction would play out if this family is on a thriving trajectory? How would it play out on a disintegrating trajectory?

3. If this family was on a disintegrating trajectory, what do you think would happen if the son got in a tough situation past curfew? How would the system respond? What would be the flexibility rules? Would you guess they would be rigid or chaotic? What would tell you whether they were one or the other?

Example #4: A Couple Talking to A Therapist About Their In-Laws

Therapist: Tell me about your relationship with your in-laws. How do you feel about them?

Partner 1: It's complicated. They can be overbearing and intrusive at times, but they also have good intentions.

Partner 2: I agree, but sometimes their good intentions come across as criticism. They just don't understand our relationship and what works for us.

Therapist: Can you give me an example of that?

Partner 1: Well, my mother-in-law always tries to give us parenting advice, even though she hasn't had young kids in a long time. It can be frustrating because she doesn't understand the challenges we face.

Partner 2: And my parents always try to get us to come over for dinner or holidays, even though we've told them multiple times that we prefer to have our own traditions and routines.

Therapist: It sounds like there are different expectations and boundaries being set here. Have you talked to your in-laws about how you feel and what you need from the relationship?

Partner 1: We've tried, but it never seems to stick. They just don't listen or understand.

Partner 2: And sometimes it feels like they're trying to come between us as a couple and our own family unit.

1. If you were this couple's therapist, what would you ask next? How would you use the EPIC framework to get the information you need to make a systemic diagnosis?
2. What questions would be important to ask this couple to make a clear statement about this system's history? How could you ask those questions in relation to the conversation that is currently taking place?
3. How might those questions be different if the identity or context of this system were different?
4. A therapist may want to try and intervene with this couple at this point. What information might the therapist miss if they started to intervene?

Example #5: A Therapist and a Teenager Talking

Therapist: How are things going with your parents?

Teenager: They're okay, I guess. But sometimes they just don't understand me.

Therapist: What do you mean by that?

Teenager: Well, they're always trying to control what I do and who I hang out with. They don't trust me to make my own decisions.

Therapist: How does that make you feel?

Teenager: Frustrated, mostly. I just want them to see that I'm capable of making good decisions for myself.

Therapist: It's natural for parents to worry about their children and want to protect them, but it's also important for teenagers to have some independence and room to make mistakes. Have you tried talking to your parents about how you feel?

Teenager: I have, but they don't seem to listen. They just say that I don't know what's best for me and that they're trying to help.

1. Given this teenager's description what questions could you ask to get a better sense of the rules of the family? What questions might help you understand the homeostasis rules? The flexibility rules?
2. What important contextual or developmental factors could you ask about? Would these help you understand the patterns? If so, how?
3. If this teenager became resistant to your questions, how else could you gather the information you need? What activities could you do? What elements could you ask to join you in session? Why would you do that?

If you've found these examples and questions to be useful, I'd encourage you to check out some of the AI platforms that are out there and ask it to generate more examples. As AI continues to generate examples and gets better at it, I recommend thinking through what you might ask next and why you would ask it. The more you do this, I think the better you will become at gathering good information and making good systemic diagnoses. As you get better at making systemic diagnoses, my hope is that you'll find that your options for intervening will grow and that you'll be better equipped to help the systems thrive.

Glossary of Terms

Adaptation   changes to the processes and interactions of a system to allow the system to maintain its autonomy

Attachment system   a system within a family system comprised of two individual elements

Autonomy   the generation and maintenance of a system through processes and interactions

Belonging process   all interactions in the family system that try to maintain connection between the elements

Biological system   any system that is autonomous and adaptable

Biomedical model   a model to understand disease that proposes that individual biological factors are the central components of health with the acknowledgement that other factors also contribute

Biopsychosocial model   a model to understand disease that proposes that illness, an individual, a family, and their social context are interconnected systems of health

Boundary   how a system distinguishes itself from the environment; a boundary is created by the separation from the environment rules of a system

Calcification   the dividing out of responsibilities of homeostasis rules to elements; for systems with disintegrating trajectories, it is the solidifying of how a system maintains stability

Communication (in social systems)   the elements of a social system; it consists of utterance, information, and understanding the difference between utterance and information

Conflict (in social systems)   the communication of contradiction; conflict in social systems occurs when communication that contradicts the dominant narrative is produced

Constitutive dimension   the stability and flexibility of processes and interactions within the systems are generated and enhanced; the structure of a system

Consubstantial   of the same substance or essence

Context   the environment or developmental niche of a system; describes the present system-environment relationship

Contradiction (in social systems)   the warning and alarm function in social systems; contradictions signal an inappropriateness of the system structures

Diagnosis (in family therapy)   the application of theory to the immediate context; a description of the system, problem, or issue based on a theory

Diagnosis   a classification of an illness or problem based on symptoms

Diagnostic process   tasks used to gather information regarding symptoms to formulate a diagnosis

Disintegrating trajectories   systems whose adaptive path results in increasingly calcified and polarized homeostasis and flexibility rules; systems in these trajectories are at risk of decreasing or losing autonomy

Elements   the components of systems that interact; things that can interact with other things

Family system   a system created by the genetic, individual, attachment, and triangulation systems

Family therapy models   collections of interventions used to address therapeutic issues

Flexibility   a system's ability to generate answers to conditions or changes in the environment

Flexibility rules   patterns in a family system that determine what types of response the system can generate in response to the environment

Genetic system   a system whose elements include genes and the epigenome

Historical dimension   details how a system has adapted and developed across time

Homeostasis rules   patterns of the threat-response, belonging, and individual interactions to try and regulate stability or maintain a constant internal environment

Individual system   a system whose elements include the cardiovascular system, the brain and nervous system, and many others; the element interactions that give rise to emotions, cognitions, and identities

Individuality process   any interaction that is the impetus for an element in a system to maintain autonomy

Interactions   create and maintain the system; the result of threat-response, individuality, and belonging processes of the elements of a system

Interactive dimension   how the system interacts with the environment; the boundary of a system

Intervention (in family therapy)   the assumed remedy for the diagnosis; what is done to change or alter the present and future of the system, problem, or issue

Medical model   the process used to advise on, coordinate, or provide intervention for improved health

Polarization   a state of a system's flexibility rules on a disintegrating trajectory; polarized flexibility rules are either rigid or chaotic

Processes   actions of elements that give rise to interactions; in a family system, three processes give rise to interactions threat-response, belonging, and individuality processes

Purpose   a system's desire to maintain its autonomy; may result in competing autonomy between elements in a system

Relational diagnosis   a model of diagnosis that aims at classifying symptoms that occur between two or more people

Resistance   perceived rigid and inflexible responses that a system gives to another system or the environment

Robustness   concerned with maintaining the possibility of a system to function rather than maintaining an actual state of a system; the steady adaptation of homeostasis rules

Rules   patterns of interactions that can become calcified or polarized

Social system   a system that sustains itself through interactions with different elements across time; social systems need new interactions and new elements to be perpetual so that they remain relevant and ongoing

Sociocultural system   the system in which the family system is embedded; comprised of social and physical environmental systems

Structure   a description of the intrinsic interactions or processes that provide stability and flexibility for the family system; the constitutive dimension of a system

System   any entity that has elements, interactions, and purpose

Systemic diagnosis   a description of the history, structure, and boundaries of a system

Theory (in family therapy)   a set of assumptions and hypotheses that predict a phenomenon and circumscribe possible explanations

Threat-response process   any interactions that occur within elements of a systems that help it respond to changes either within the system or the environment

Thriving trajectory   adaptation pathways that are marked by robust and flexible homeostasis and flexibility rules

Triangulation system   a system within the family system that is comprised of interactions between overlapping attachment systems

Working diagnosis   one or more potential diagnoses that are confirmed or discarded based on treatment response and additional information gathering

References

Afifi, T. D., Merrill, A. F., & Davis, S. (2016). The theory of resilience and relational load. *Personal Relationships*, *23*(4), 663–683.

Allen, K. R., & Henderson, A. C. (2016). *Family theories: Foundations and applications*. John Wiley & Sons.

Baldwin, D., Woods, R., Lawson, R., & Taylor, D. (2011). Efficacy of drug treatments for generalized anxiety disorder: Systematic review and meta-analysis. *BMJ*, *342*.

Baraldi, C., Corsi, G., & Esposito, E. (2021). Unlocking Luhmann. In *Unlocking Luhmann*. Bielefeld University Press, transcript.

Bekar, C., & Lipsey, R. G. (2004). Science, institutions and the industrial revolution. *Journal of European Economic History*, *33*(3), 709–753.

Bender, S., Stokes, A., & Gaspaire, S. (2018). Implications of the coverage of the" DSM-5" in textbooks on learning and teaching of psychology within higher education. *Psychology Teaching Review*, *24*(1), 53–58.

Bertalanffy, L. V. (1968). *General system theory: Foundations, development, applications*. G. Braziller.

Blashfield, R. K., Keeley, J. W., Flanagan, E. H., & Miles, S. R. (2014). The cycle of classification: DSM-I through DSM-5. *Annual Review of Clinical Psychology*, *10*, 25–51.

Caldwell, B. E., Woolley, S. R., & Caldwell, C. J. (2007). Preliminary estimates of cost-effectiveness for marital therapy. *Journal of Marital and Family Therapy*, *33*(3), 392–405.

Carcone, D., & Ruocco, A. C. (2017). Six years of research on the national institute of mental health's research domain criteria (RDoC) initiative: A systematic review. *Frontiers in Cellular Neuroscience*, *11*, 46.

Carr, A. (2015). The evolution of systems theory. In *Handbook of family therapy* (pp. 13–29). Routledge.

Chen, R., Hughes, A. C., & Austin, J. P. (2017). The use of theory in family therapy research: Content analysis and update. *Journal of Marital and Family Therapy*, *43*(3), 514–525.

Chmielewski, M., Clark, L. A., Bagby, R. M., & Watson, D. (2015). Method matters: Understanding diagnostic reliability in DSM-IV and DSM-5. *Journal of Abnormal Psychology*, *124*(3), 764.

Clarke, D. E., Narrow, W. E., Regier, D. A., Kuramoto, S. J., Kupfer, D. J., Kuhl, E. A., . . . Kraemer, H. C. (2013). DSM-5 field trials in the United States and Canada, part I: Study design, sampling strategy, implementation, and analytic approaches. *American Journal of Psychiatry, 170*(1), 43–58.

Clawson, R. E., Davis, S. Y., Miller, R. B., & Webster, T. N. (2018). The case for insurance reimbursement of couple therapy. *Journal of Marital and Family Therapy, 44*(3), 512–526.

Clegg, J. W. (2012). Teaching about mental health and illness through the history of the DSM. *History of Psychology, 15*(4), 364.

Cosgrove, L., Krimsky, S., Vijayaraghavan, M., & Schneider, L. (2006). Financial ties between DSM-IV panel members and the pharmaceutical industry. *Psychotherapy and Psychosomatics, 75*(3), 154–160.

Cuijpers, P., Stringaris, A., & Wolpert, M. (2020). Treatment outcomes for depression: Challenges and opportunities. *The Lancet Psychiatry, 7*(11), 925–927.

Cuijpers, P., & van Straten, A. (2014). Improving outcomes in social anxiety disorder. *The Lancet Psychiatry, 1*(5), 324–326.

Cuthbert, B. N., & Insel, T. R. (2013). Toward the future of psychiatric diagnosis: The seven pillars of RDoC. *BMC Medicine, 11*(1), 1–8.

Denton, W., & Coalition Members. (1989). *Rationale for the inclusion of relational disorders with DSM-IV.* Coalition on Family Diagnosis.

Engel, G. L. (1977). The need for a new medical model: A challenge for biomedicine. *Science, 196*(4286), 129–136.

Frances, A. (2012). *DSM-5 field trials discredit the American psychiatric association.* www.huffpost.com/entry/dsm-5-field-trials-discre_b_2047621

Guillory, P. T. (2021). *Emotionally focused therapy with African American couples: Love heals.* Routledge.

Guy, J. S. (2018). Is Niklas Luhmann a relational sociologist? *The Palgrave Handbook of Relational Sociology,* 289–304.

Hartman IV, J. L., Garvik, B., & Hartwell, L. (2001). Principles for the buffering of genetic variation. *Science, 291*(5506), 1001–1004.

Hayes, S. C., & Hofmann, S. G. (Eds.). (2020). *Beyond the DSM: Toward a process-based alternative for diagnosis and mental health treatment.* New Harbinger Publications.

Hill, C. E., Spiegel, S. B., Hoffman, M. A., Kivlighan Jr, D. M., & Gelso, C. J. (2017). Therapist expertise in psychotherapy revisited. *The Counseling Psychologist, 45*(1), 7–53.

Holt-Lunstad, J., Smith, T. B., & Layton, J. B. (2010). Social relationships and mortality risk: A meta-analytic review. *PLoS Medicine, 7*(7), e1000316.

Huda, A. S. (2019). *The medical model in mental health: An explanation and evaluation.* Oxford University Press.

Jutel, A. (2009). Sociology of diagnosis: A preliminary review. *Sociology of Health and Illness, 31*(2), 278–299.

Kangan, N. H. (2020). The critical relationship between anxiety and depression. *American Journal of Psychiatry, 177*(5), 365–367.

Kaslow, F. W. (1996). *Handbook of relational diagnosis and dysfunctional family patterns.* John Wiley & Sons.

Kerr, M. E., & Bowen, M. (1988). *Family evaluation.* WW Norton & Company.

Kessler, R. C., Avenevoli, S., Costello, E. J., Georgiades, K., Green, J. G., Gruber, M. J., . . . Merikangas, K. R. (2012). Prevalence, persistence, and sociodemographic correlates of DSM-IV disorders in the national comorbidity survey replication adolescent supplement. *Archives of General Psychiatry, 69*(4), 372–380.

Kessler, R. C., Chiu, W. T., Demler, O., & Walters, E. E. (2005). Prevalence, severity, and comorbidity of 12-month DSM-IV disorders in the national comorbidity survey replication. *Archives of General Psychiatry, 62*(6), 617–627.

Kline, A. C., Cooper, A. A., Rytwinski, N. K., & Feeny, N. C. (2021). The effect of concurrent depression on PTSD outcomes in trauma-focused psychotherapy: A meta-analysis of randomized controlled trials. *Behavior Therapy, 52*(1), 250–266.

Law, D. D., & Crane, D. R. (2000). The influence of marital and family therapy on health care utilization in a health-maintenance organization. *Journal of Marital and Family Therapy, 26*(3), 281–291.

Lebow, J. (2015). Relational diagnosis-an idea whose time has come. *Family Process, 54*(1), 1–5.

Lebow, J., & Gordon, K. C. (2006). You cannot choose what is not on the menu – Obstacles to and reasons for the inclusion of relational processes in the DSM-V: Comment on the special section. *Journal of Family Psychology, 20*(3), 432.

Luhmann, N. (1984). *Social systems.* Stanford University Press.

McCarthy, J. (2022). *Same-sex marriage support inches up to new high of 71%.* Gallup. https://news.gallup.com/poll/393197/same-sex-marriage-support-inches-new-high.aspx

Meadows, D. H. (2008). *Thinking in systems: A primer.* Chelsea Green Publishing.

Moreno, A., & Mossio, M. (2015). *Biological autonomy.* A Philo.

National Academies of Sciences, Engineering, and Medicine. (2015). *Improving diagnosis in health care.* National Academies Press.

Negash, S., Chung, K., & Oh, S. (2022). Families post-release: Barriers and pathways to family therapy. *Family Process, 61*(2), 609–624.

Ngo, M., Rauffet, P., & Banks, S. (2022). Exploring multitasking performance and fatigue with the MATB-II: A narrative. *Human Error, Reliability, Resilience, and Performance, 33*, 22.

Oyama, S. (2000). *The ontogeny of information: Developmental systems and evolution.* Duke University Press.

Plana-Ripoll, O., Pedersen, C. B., Holtz, Y., Benros, M. E., Dalsgaard, S., De Jonge, P., . . . McGrath, J. J. (2019). Exploring comorbidity within mental disorders among a Danish national population. *JAMA Psychiatry, 76*(3), 259–270.

Priest, J. B. (2021). *The science of family systems theory.* Routledge.

Reiter, M. D. (2016). A quick guide to case conceptualization in structural family therapy. *Journal of Systemic Therapies, 35*(2), 25–37.

Ross, C. A., & Margolis, R. L. (2019). Research domain criteria: Strengths, weaknesses, and potential alternatives for future psychiatric research. *Complex Psychiatry, 5*(4), 218–236.

Rosslenbroich, B. (2014). *On the origin of autonomy: A new look at the major transitions in evolution* (Vol. 5). Springer Science & Business Media.

Shah, P., & Mountain, D. (2007). The medical model is dead – long live the medical model. *The British Journal of Psychiatry, 191*(5), 375–377.

Shorter, E. (2015). *What psychiatry left out of the DSM-5: Historical mental disorders today.* Routledge.

Snyder, D. K., Heyman, R. E., Haynes, S. N., Carlson, C. I., & Balderrama-Durbin, C. (2019). Couple and family assessment. In *APA handbook of contemporary family psychology: Family therapy and training* (Vol. 3, pp. 35–51). American Psychological Association.

Sperry, L. (2005). Case conceptualization: A strategy for incorporating individual, couple and family dynamics in the treatment process. *The American Journal of Family Therapy, 33*(5), 353–364.

Touboul, P., Métris, G., Rodrigues, M., Bergé, J., Robert, A., Baghi, Q., . . . & Visser, P. (2022). MICROSCOPE mission: Final results of the test of the equivalence principle. *Physical Review Letters, 129*(12), 121102.

Tuggy, D. (2013). *Trinity.* Lulu. Com.

University of Chicago. (1896). *Annual register July, 1895–July, 1896 with announcements for 1896-7.* University of Chicago Press. www.google.com/books/edition/Annual_Register_with_Announcements_for/HysXAAAAYAAJ?hl=en&gbpv=0

Vaidyanathan, U., Morris, S., Wagner, A., Sherrill, J., Sommers, D., Garvey, M., Murphy, E., & Cuthbert, B. (2020). The NIHM research domain criteria project. In S. G. Hoffman & S. C. Hayes (Eds.), *Beyond the DSM: Toward a process-based alternative for diagnosis and mental health treatment.* New Harbinger Publications.

Wamboldt, M., Cordaro Jr., A., & Clarke, D. (2015). Parent – child relational problem: Field trial results, changes in DSM-5, and proposed changes for ICD-11. *Family Process, 54*(1), 33–47.

Weber, M. (2002). *The protestant ethic and the spirit of capitalism: And other writings.* Penguin.

Wittenborn, A. K., & Holtrop, K. (2022). Introduction to the special issue on the efficacy and effectiveness of couple and family interventions: Evidence base update 2010–2019. *Journal of Marital and Family Therapy, 48*(1), 5–22.

Wittenborn, A. K., Woods, S. B., Priest, J. B., Morgan, P. C., Tseng, C. F., Huerta, P., & Edwards, C. (2022). Couple and family interventions for depressive and bipolar disorders: Evidence base update (2010–2019). *Journal of Marital and Family Therapy, 48*(1), 129–153.

Woods, S. B. (2019). Biopsychosocial theories. In *APA handbook of contemporary family psychology: Foundations, methods, and contemporary issues across the lifespan* (Vol. 1, pp. 75–92). American Psychological Association.

Yang, Y. C., Boen, C., Gerken, K., Li, T., Schorpp, K., & Harris, K. M. (2016). Social relationships and physiological determinants of longevity across the human life span. *Proceedings of the National Academy of Sciences, 113*(3), 578–583.

Index

Note: Page numbers in *italics* indicate a figure on the corresponding page.